Praise fo
Yoga and Vega...

"In *Yoga and Veganism*, Sharon Gannon radiates timeless wisdom and applies ancient truths to contemporary customs. She describes how yoga and a vegan diet can help heal our society's 'disease of disconnection' and remedies a mind-set that has allowed cruelty and violence to become normalized on our troubled planet. I hope everybody will read Sharon's book, which describes how our actions affect our world and how we can liberate ourselves through compassion to others."
—GENE BAUR, founder of Farm Sanctuary

"If we are to survive as a species, we need to improve our relationships with animals and nature; this book will show you how."
—DUNCAN WONG, founder of Yogic Arts

"Reading *Yoga and Veganism* . . . I was enchanted, challenged, and moved. This beautiful book reminds us that loving-kindness is at the heart of yoga."
—KAREN DAWN, founder of DawnWatch and author of
Thanking the Monkey: Rethinking the Way We Treat Animals

"Sharon's mission of *ahimsa* is so deep and profound; she writes from her heart and soul."
—GURMUKH KAUR KHALSA, director of Golden Bridge Yoga

"Sharon Gannon's commitment to animal rights has been evident in every aspect of her life. She recognizes that the continued murder and slavery of animals affects all levels of consciousness, as well as our health, environment, and global famine, and that it will only be through individual shifts of mindfulness that this suffering can finally end. A modern, compassionate, and well-informed voice for Self-realization and planetary change, she has been unwavering in her quest to educate humankind that our animal brothers and sisters are experiencing a mass level of intolerable abuse that must be addressed if we believe in creating a world that is sustainable, harmonious, and peaceful for all. In her new book, Sharon uses the traditional text of Patanjali's Yoga Sutras to draw our awareness to how our actions affect each other and the world we share. I highly recommend this informative book as an excellent resource to anyone interested in understanding yoga, its principles, and how these ancient teachings can impact all beings and species in these contemporary and complicated times."

—SEANE CORN, yoga teacher, co-founder of Off the Mat, Into the World and author of *Revolution of the Soul: Awaken to Love Through Raw Truth, Radical Healing, and Conscious Action*

"Sharon's writing is born from her commitment to walking the talk. She is the living embodiment of the selflessness she teaches and has had a profound impact on my life as a musician and peace worker. She encourages me by her example to mean what I say and to say what I mean with each breath and with every smile."

—MICHAEL FRANTI, musician, activist, and author of *Food for the Masses: Lyrics & Portraits*

"Sharon Gannon beautifully illustrates the perfect symbiosis of yoga and veganism. The most mindful, spiritual, soulful practice married to the most healthful, harmless, life-affirming diet—what could be more intuitive, more beneficial, and more necessary?"

—RORY FREEDMAN, co-author of the #1 *New York Times* best seller *Skinny Bitch*

"A prayer as pledge, a practice opening compassion, a yoke that gives freedom, a strength that comes from kindness, a yoga book that reveals how beautifully liberating animal-free eating is."

—CAROL J. ADAMS, author of *The Sexual Politics of Meat: A Feminist-Vegetarian Critical Theory* and co-author of *Protest Kitchen: Fight Injustice, Save the Planet, and Fuel Your Resistance One Meal at a Time*

"The urgency of ahimsa and animal protection, especially when it comes to our own diets, is a very important component of spiritual life, and is often underestimated. Few have been as outspoken on this as Sharon Gannon, who has written a pioneering, groundbreaking work on this subject. It is innovative and important because through her insightful investigation of the yogic scriptures she has taken the subject to new depths, going beyond the common conception of ahimsa and showing how universal compassion manifests in satya, asteya, brahmacharya, and aparigraha as well. She also reveals the connection between asana and veganism—perhaps for the first time—and also how a compassionate vegan diet intersects with Patanjali's kriya yoga (tapas, svadhyaya, and ishvarapranidhana). In other words, her book should be considered *the* guidebook on the yoga of action or modern-day spiritual activism. Indeed, she is to be applauded for her efforts on behalf of ourselves, the planet, and our four-footed, scaly, and feathered kin."

    —STEVEN J. ROSEN (SATYARAJA DASA), biographer, scholar, and author in the fields of philosophy, Indic religion, and comparative spirituality

"*Sarve Sukhino Bhavantu*: "May all beings be happy." This is the universal message of true spirituality. Compassion to all beings is the natural expression of one who is spiritually awakened. To be an instrument of God's love in all that we do is an essential practice and the goal of yoga. In *Yoga and Veganism*, Sharon Gannon shares the treasures of her own compassionate heart, and her lifetime of study and practice. In doing so, she helps us to connect with our own hearts and the hearts of all life-loving beings. I am sincerely grateful to Sharon for her genuine kindness and for this illuminating book."

    —H. H. RADHANATH SWAMI, spiritual leader, activist, and best-selling author of *The Journey Home: Autobiography of an American Swami* and *The Journey Within: Exploring the Path of Bhakti*

"Yoga means *connection*, but yoga is much more than uniting with one's physical body. Through bhakti yoga, loving devotion to God, a soulful bond is established with the Divine presence. Entering into such a relationship with the Supreme requires a body, mind, and heart that has been purified and is maintained through a sattvic vegan diet. As described in this book, veganism will bring the practitioner closer to *mukti*, that state of eternal bliss and total love."

    —SHRI MILAN GOSWAMI, spiritual leader, direct descendant and lineage holder of the Pushti Marg (Path of Grace) Sampradaya of Vallabhacharya

Also by
SHARON GANNON

Freedom Is a Psycho-Kinetic Skill (1982)

Cats and Dogs Are People Too! (1999)
(Italian-language translation available)

*Jivamukti Yoga: Practices for Liberating Body
and Soul* (with David Life) (2002)
(German, Italian, Russian, and Spanish translations available)

The Art of Yoga (with David Life) (2002)

Jivamukti Yoga Chant Book (2003)
(Chinese, French, German, Italian, Japanese, Russian,
Spanish, and Turkish translations available)

Yoga and Vegetarianism (2008)
(Chinese, German, Italian, Japanese, Russian,
Spanish, and Turkish translations available)

*Yoga Assists: A Complete Visual and Inspirational Guide
to Yoga Asana Assists* (with David Life) (2013)
(Italian translation available)

*Simple Recipes for Joy: More Than 200
Delicious Vegan Recipes* (2014)
(Italian translation available)

*The Magic Ten and Beyond: Daily Spiritual Practice
for Greater Peace and Well-Being* (2018)
(Italian translation available)

The Art of Norahs Nepas (2019)

YOGA &

VEGANISM

The Diet of Enlightenment

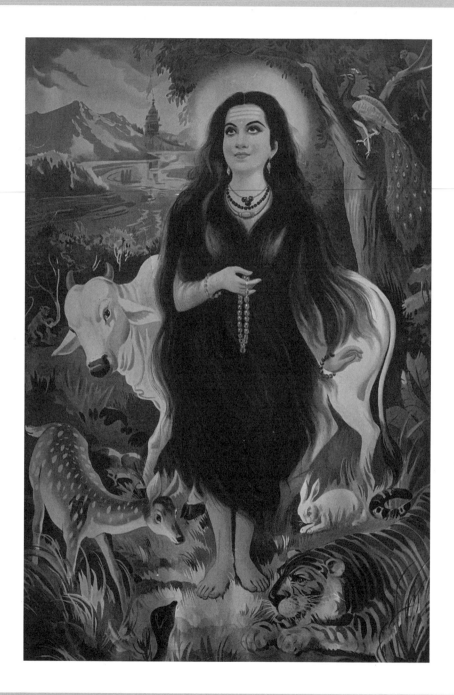

YOGA &
VEGANISM

The Diet of Enlightenment

Practical Activism for Global
and Personal Transformation

SHARON GANNON

Foreword by Ingrid Newkirk

MANDALA

San Rafael • Los Angeles • London

MANDALA

An Imprint of MandalaEarth
PO Box 3088
San Rafael, CA 94912
www.MandalaEarth.com

 Find us on Facebook: www.facebook.com/
MandalaEarth
Follow us on Twitter: @MandalaEarth

JIVAMUKTI YOGA®
www.jivamuktiyoga.com

Library of Congress Cataloging-in-Publication Data available.

ISBN: 978-1-68383-922-4

Publisher: Raoul Goff
President: Kate Jerome
Associate Publisher: Phillip Jones
Design Support: Malea Clark-Nicholson
Managing Editor: Lauren LePera
Senior Production Manager: Greg Steffen

The content of this book is provided for informational purposes only and is not intended to diagnose, treat, or cure any conditions without the assistance of a trained practitioner. If you are experiencing a medical condition, seek care from an appropriate licensed professional.

The essays featured in the "Transformational Stories" chapter are used by permission of the respective author. Foreword by Ingrid Newkirk used by permission.

"Chocolate Layer Cake," "Vanilla Sugar Icing," "Spirulina Millet," and "'Poached Eggs' on Toast" from SIMPLE RECIPES FOR JOY: MORE THAN 200 DELICIOUS VEGAN RECIPES by Sharon Gannon, copyright © 2014 by Sharon Gannon. Used by permission of Penguin Books, an imprint of Penguin Publishing Group, a division of Penguin Random House LLC. All rights reserved.

Grateful acknowledgment to the following individuals for their work on the original edition of *Yoga and Vegetarianism*: Iain R. Morris, Jake Gerli, Arjuna van der Kooij, Lucy Kee, Leslie Cohen, Mary Teruel, Lallo Lemos.

The image on page 6 depicts Akka Mahadevi (12th century), a medieval female saint and poet from South India with an unusually modern outlook, venerated as a symbol of the equality of women and as an early exponent of women's emancipation, environmentalism, vegetarianism, and animal rights. She lived in the forest with wild animals, birds, trees, and flowers as her friends. She rejected marriage and family life and chose God as her eternal husband. A true ascetic, Akka Mahadevi is said to have refused to wear any clothing (using only her long hair for coverage), a common practice among male ascetics, but shocking for a woman.

Photograph of the author on page 199 by Derek Pashupa Goodwin.

This book is printed on recycled paper meeting the strictest requirements to ensure sustainable forests. The recycled fibers are processed in a chlorine-free process (TCF). TCF bleaching is a pollution prevention process that does not create dioxins in our waterways or air.

ROOTS of PEACE   REPLANTED PAPER

Mandala Publishing, in association with Roots of Peace, will plant two trees for each tree used in the manufacturing of this book. Roots of Peace is an internationally renowned humanitarian organization dedicated to eradicating land mines worldwide and converting war-torn lands into productive farms and wildlife habitats. Roots of Peace will plant two million fruit and nut trees in Afghanistan and provide farmers there with the skills and support necessary for sustainable land use.

Manufactured in India by Insight Editions

10 9 8 7 6 5 4 3 2 1

To those who want to be free
To those who do not want to be hurt by others
To those who do not want to be lied to—
who want to be listened to
To those who do not want to live in poverty
To those who want to be healthy and well
To those who want to know the purpose of their lives

This book is dedicated to you, the people of this planet Earth,
the citizens of this universe, present and future.

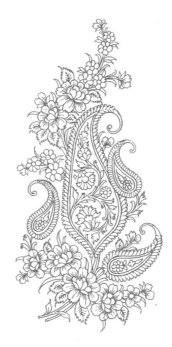

CONTENTS

A Note on the Text

Originally published as *Yoga and Vegetarianism*, this updated edition has been expanded with additional material, including a revised introduction, a new chapter featuring essays from individuals whose lives have been transformed by veganism—including Ingrid Newkirk (president of the People for the Ethical Treatment of Animals, or PETA), Kip Andersen (award-winning filmmaker), Victoria Moran (founder of the Main Street Vegan Academy), and others—a supplementary chapter containing vegan recipes from the author, an expanded Q&A section and resources list, and an index for easy reference.

Throughout the book, the following conventions are used with regard to the words *yoga* and *self*: An uppercase *Y* is used when referring to *Yoga* as a state of enlightenment, and a lowercase *y* is used in *yoga* when referring to yoga practices. An uppercase *S* is used when referring to the larger concept of Self, which is eternal and all-inclusive, and a lowercase *s* is used to refer to the self as it pertains to the individual ego.

A Note on Sanskrit Transliteration

The chants from the yoga scriptures are spelled using the transliteration guide set forth below. The pronunciation examples are based on American English.

a	cut	i	pit	U	pull	e	say	o	cone
ā	father	ī	seek	Ū	soon	ai	pile	au	now

ḥ: slight aspiration or echo of the preceding syllable (as in the word *namaḥ*, which is pronounced with slight breath of air at the end as *namaha*)

ṁ: the nasal sound in the French word *bon*; sometimes pronounced like the English "m"

ṇ: *nice*, but with the tongue curled up against the palate

ś: a "sh" sound, as in *shine*

ṣ: the "sh" sound above, but with the tongue curled up against the palate

ṭ: a "t" sound, as in *time*, but with the tongue curled up against the palate

ṭh: pronounced as a separate "t" and "h" in close succession, as in *account holder*, but with the tongue curled up against the palate (aspirated ṭ)

FOREWORD

by Ingrid Newkirk

IN 2008, HIS HOLINESS THE DALIA LAMA, ONE OF THE most enlightened souls among us, who has lived under threat of attack and death for most of his years, wrote, "Kindness is my religion."

Although His Holiness has experienced more persecution than most, he is certainly not the first great thinker to recognize the overwhelming value of compassion. In the 1800s, the celebrated British writer Henry James proclaimed that there are three things in life that count: "The first is to be kind," he wrote. The second is to be kind. And, yes, as you've no doubt guessed, the third is to be kind.

Kindness is the magic word that links, with all-encompassing positivism, every being in the universe to all the others. Through meditation and self-awareness, yogis come to see this interconnectedness that most of humanity only dreams of, yet there are clear and easy steps all "mere mortals" can take to reach this understanding.

Sharon Gannon, the author of this life-guidance book, knows and teaches the vital role of kindness in expanding our spiritual horizons and shaping our personal and collective history. She is one of the kindest people I have ever met, and her deep love for others of all kinds—from mouse to man, from the starving child to the superstar—not only shines through her eyes but also seems to radiate through her very skin. She has that luminescence that comes from inner peace. Her petite frame belies a powerful spirit with the ability—so often lost in the blur of modern life—to empathize with others, *all* others, whether familiars or strangers, and with all the vast animal nations, including our own.

Sharon chose to become a yoga teacher at a time when yoga was viewed by most as a trendy form of physical fitness. She has endured the skepticism of her peers and colleagues in her unapologetic commitment to teaching yoga as a means to enlightenment through compassion for all beings. She has infused her now very popular method of yoga with a strong animal rights and vegan message. Her scholarly understanding of the Sanskrit language and the Yoga Sutras has allowed her to cite yogic scriptural references to support her defense of animals as worthy of our compassion and care. At first, her critics told her she was too extreme to bring her own political views and dietary preferences into the classroom. However, she persevered—as all great, radical activists have always done—and has made enduring changes in the way that many yoga practitioners, as well as ordinary people, view animals and themselves. She knows and teaches that true spiritual development can happen only through actively extending kindness to all beings.

Sharon learned from her animal friends and protectors when she was just a tot. Humanity is still learning but is often only entertained—rather than enlightened—by the newspaper accounts of studies showing that all living beings are marvelously inspiring and can teach us much about how to live, how to react, and how to cope if we open our eyes.

It is indisputable that all other animals (for we are but one) share our capacity for love, grief, joy, and pain. Once upon a time, we ruled the Earth with an iron fist, taking whatever we desired from anyone and everyone powerless to defend themselves, including people of other colors and abilities, and it was acceptable to treat animals as inanimate objects. Today, unless we have hardened our hearts and closed our minds to reason, we appreciate them as sentient forms of diverse life, as the "spirits" that they are. We see that we are surrounded by "others" whose lives are interwoven with ours, and we realize that whether they live at the bottom of our garden or are flying over our heads, animals treasure their freedom as much as and as passionately as we do ours.

As Sharon makes clear, animals are no threat to us; rather, they are our neighbors and allies. Accepting them helps us grow closer to the oneness of life. As philosopher Henry Beston wrote, "We need another and a wiser and perhaps a more mystical concept of animals. . . . We patronize them for their incompleteness, for their tragic fate of having taken form so far below ourselves. And therein we err, and greatly err. For the animal shall not be measured by man. In a world older and more complete than ours, they move finished and complete, gifted with extensions of the senses that we have lost or never attained, living by voices we shall never hear. They are not brethren, they are not underlings; they are other nations caught with ourselves in the net of life and time, fellow prisoners of the splendor and travail of the Earth."

Through her personal stories and insight, Sharon draws us into other worlds. She reminds us *who* animals are. Elephants weep for beloved lost relatives, prairie dogs use nouns, crows not only use but also make tools, mice giggle, cows give a little jump for joy when they solve a puzzle, and birds seek medicinal clay to treat their wounds. She awakens us to the fact that all beings communicate: Rhinoceroses use breath language, dolphins converse perhaps by sending whole pictures, cows recognize their fellows' almost invisible facial movements, frogs use vibrations to drum messages to one another, a squid can flirt with another squid to his left and fend off a squid to his right by creating a message using different waves and patterns of colors on either side of his body, and birds sing at frequencies and speeds too high and fast for us to hear unless we capture the sounds with sophisticated equipment and slow down the recordings.

Sharon helps us see that play, a sophisticated concept, is a delight throughout the animal nations, too: It is not only wild cats and dogs or domesticated ones who roll about with retracted claws and play-bite for fun and tease one another. She asks us to see that we share with the other animals not only emotions but also all manner of traits and abilities once thought to be unique to the physically able white man—then only to humans. For instance, fish tell time, octopuses move their finds about on the walls of their dens until they have decorated to their liking, jays play tricks on one another, deer will risk their own lives to stay with an injured mate, and chickens will turn the heater up in their barn on a cold morning if given the opportunity to do so.

These are only a few among countless examples of animals' interests and feelings. Knowing this, we must find it within ourselves, particularly as we strive to be better people, to cast off all hatred, prejudice, and selfishness and to embrace animals as our fellows. Animals are individuals with families who are traveling through life, as we are, vulnerable and hopeful, like us vested with dreams and the desire to escape suffering. This book opens our eyes and hearts to the beautiful prospect of being a far bigger part of life—not apart from life—and finding on Earth the very thing our space programs seek elsewhere: connection with intelligent forms of life.

We go through life having many lessons to learn, and those of us who seek to be better people try hard to mold ourselves into beings we can be pleased about, spiritually successful, able to conquer our base desires, and striving to be virtuous. By working to extend our kindness to all, without bias and without asking for anything in return, we realize our own potential as good people.

INGRID NEWKIRK is the founder and president of People for the Ethical Treatment of Animals (PETA) and the author of Making Kind Choices *and co-author of* One Can Make a Difference.

PROLOGUE

YOGA STUDENTS OFTEN ASK ME, "WHAT DOES PRACTICING yoga have to do with veganism?" I hope to answer that question in this book by exploring Patanjali's Yoga Sutras, a scriptural text he compiled over a thousand years ago that lays out the philosophical underpinnings of yoga.

I became a yoga teacher only because I felt it might provide a platform for me to speak out for animal rights. I was hopeful that I might be able to somehow contribute to the evolution of human consciousness so that we, as a species, could begin to see ourselves as holy—as part of a whole.

Some people call themselves animal rights activists yet believe that it is permissible to use animals—and even eat them—provided that they are given a nice life before being killed. I, on the other hand, can see no way in which the exploitation of animals for our own selfish needs is ever permissible. When it comes to these practices, I am an abolitionist.

In Patanjali's ancient scripture, I found the means to articulate—in a compassionate, joyful, and nonjudgmental way—a logical argument in defense of our fellow earthlings, the other animals with whom we share this phenomenal world. Patanjali's words are not only relevant to our present time but also essential for our collective future.

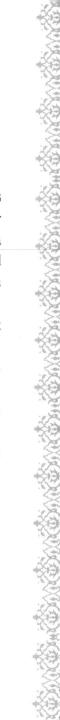

In the Yoga Sutras, Patanjali presents an eight-step plan for liberation called Raja yoga. The first step is *yama*, which means restraint. It consists of five ethical guidelines regarding how yogis should treat others, all of which clearly support a vegan diet. The first *yama* Patanjali gives is *ahimsa*, or nonharming. Patanjali implies that if we can become firmly established in ahimsa, others will cease to harm us. Many spiritual leaders have noted that there is so much suffering in the world because there is so much violence. If we can reduce the violence, we can reduce the suffering. Patanjali says future suffering should be avoided, and he prescribes *ahimsa* as the method—if we stop perpetuating violence, it will cease. If we could remain enveloped in this state of peace, we really wouldn't need to do any other yoga practice. But Patanjali recognized how rare it is for a person to be truly established in ahimsa, so he was kind enough to leave us a few more instructions!

Billions of animals are killed every year for human consumption after living confined in horrible conditions on factory farms and enduring untold extremes of suffering. This fact alone is good reason for any yoga practitioner to adopt a vegan diet. Meanwhile, from the individual health perspective, a vegan diet has been proven to prevent and even reverse heart disease[1] and cancer,[2] two of the leading causes of human death in our world today. The terrible toll that eating meat,

---

1 John Robbins, *The Food Revolution: How Your Diet Can Help Save Your Life and Our World* (Berkeley: Conari, 2001), 19.

2 American Institute for Cancer Research and World Cancer Research Fund, *Food, Nutrition, and the Prevention of Cancer: A Global Perspective* (American Institute for Cancer Research, 1997), 456–57.

fish, and dairy takes on our planet's air, water, soil, and whole ecosystem is another reason for yogis, who have traditionally cultivated a close relationship with nature, to consider veganism. Finally, as yogis, our ultimate goal is enlightenment, which involves realizing the unity and interconnectedness of *all* beings and things—not just human beings. Extending compassion toward animals purifies our karmas, creating an internal state that is conducive to enlightenment.

My own journey to becoming a vegan animal rights activist yoga teacher began when I was three years old. I lived in Florida with my mother, father, little brother, and my friend, Mrs. Goose. My parents referred to Mrs. Goose as my "imaginary friend." I did not know what that meant at the time. In my mind, Mrs. Goose was a goose only a few inches taller than I was. We all lived in a big rented house at the edge of the Everglade forest.

One day as we were returning home from the grocery store, Mrs. Goose and I wanted to race each other to the front door, and as we ran out of the car, we both spotted something colorful lying on the stone porch steps. Mrs. Goose told me to slow down and be very quiet. She waddled closer to take a look, then told me to approach quietly. As I got closer, the shiny black, red, and yellow being who was lying on the steps, bathing in the sun, opened her eyes wide to look at us. I had never seen such a creature. She lifted her head to speak. She spoke in such a low whisper that I had to lean down very near to her face to hear her.

She was just about to tell me something when I heard my mother screaming behind me. My mother came quickly, pushed Mrs. Goose out of the way, and grabbed me. My dad came running with a crowbar and hit the shiny lady, breaking her back. I heard her scream, and I tried to get free from my mother to run and help her. Mrs. Goose was doing her best to interfere by flapping her wings and squawking.

My dad hit the lady again, this time breaking her body into two pieces. My mother let me go. I ran to see the beautiful, shiny creature lying lifeless in the sun, one eye still gleaming open, looking at me. As the wind moved through the cypress trees, I heard her whisper, "Why?"

Without intending to, I had caused the death of a beautiful coral snake minding her own business, sunning herself. It was then that I realized I had the power to influence the actions of other people, for better or for worse, and I had better be careful.

I went to a Catholic school from first to sixth grade. Every morning, the day began with a catechism lesson. In first grade, we learned the Ten Commandments. The day that we learned *Thou shalt not kill,* I came home from school and was excited to tell my mother that we aren't supposed to kill. She was fixing a dish for dinner she called peasant stew, which had cut-up hot dogs in it. I knew that hamburgers and hot dogs were animals who were killed so that we could eat them, so I was very excited to tell her the news. She responded, "Don't worry. It's okay that we kill *these* animals, because they are raised for it." I went off by myself to think about this statement.

I felt very confused. I had only recently heard the story of Hansel and Gretel and the witch who fattens them up, intending to pop them in the oven and eat them for dinner. I felt bewildered, angry, and disturbed that my mother did not see the connection. I felt even more disturbed because I wasn't able to communicate to her that there seemed to be something very wrong with what we were doing. I realized that if my mother was going to change her behavior, I had to be able to communicate to her in a way that did not make her angry, and for that to happen, I couldn't be angry myself. I had to find a better way.

Years later, in 1982, while living in Seattle as a thirty-one-year-old dancer, poet, musician, and painter, I went to see *The Animals Film*—a British documentary that probed into the relationship between human beings and animals. I went because the soundtrack was by Robert Wyatt, a musician I admired. Academy Award–winning actress Julie Christie narrated the film.

Those two hours and twenty minutes in the movie theater altered my life like no other single incident. The film exposed the cruel, exploitative, and inhumane way that we human beings treat animals. The film explored the use of animals as entertainment (from stuffed toys to pets), as food, as providers of clothing, and as victims of military and "scientific" research. It ended with the Animal Liberation Front (ALF) rescuing animals from a laboratory. The movie caused me to radically rethink art, the purpose of the artist, and what I was doing with my life. If I wasn't contributing to stopping the insanity I saw depicted in this film, what was the value in what I was doing?

I had been an on-again, off-again vegetarian before the film. After viewing it, I became a committed vegetarian and, soon after, a vegan. I was deeply affected and vowed that I would find a way to help stop the suffering of the animals I had seen in the film—but how? I tried to voice my feelings, but my friends accused me of being too emotional. It was like trying to talk to my mother all over again. I knew that what I had seen was a glimpse into reality that not many people had experienced or cared to experience. I could no longer live in a cushioned state of denial. I knew that for the situation to change, a whole society had to change—indeed, a whole culture. But first, could there be a change among my circle of friends? Could *I* change? I felt incredibly inadequate and inarticulate.

While in this state of intense internal turmoil, I fell down some steep, slippery stairs and fractured my fifth lumbar vertebra. The accident resulted in paralysis of my right leg for a painful and frightening two weeks. I recovered the use of my leg, but on occasion, I would still lose all sensation when the bone shifted and pinched a nerve. During this time, I moved to New York City. My back was still injured, and I began attending yoga classes as a last-ditch effort to do something nonsurgical about the pain. Yoga not only helped my back but also instigated a reintegration of all parts of my being.

During those first few yoga classes, I had the rare experience of going deeper into the feelings in my body as well as the judgments, assumptions, and opinions in my mind. Was it painful? Extremely!

But, perhaps for the first time in my very physical life, I was actually being physical. I wasn't trying to get out of my body—I was actually going deeper into it with a sense of adventure.

Previously, as an artist and activist, I had objectified my body, considering it to be a tool I needed. After all, I was going to change the world, save the animals, and bring peace on Earth—and I needed a body to accomplish this great work!

I realized through the practice of yoga that ideas were not enough to change the world or to change my own life. Whatever I wanted to see in the world around me had to first become real in my own life, in my own body, down to the molecular level. Change had to start with the way I lived, the way I breathed, and how I spoke. Yoga gave me the means to dehypnotize myself from the cultural conditioning to which I—and everyone—had been subjected. Yoga taught me that the disease of disconnection that causes us to say one thing while meaning another—and many times, do a completely different, third thing—stems from a deep lack of self-confidence. Yoga taught me the unifying power of well-being, which arises through aligning with breath (the animating life force) and allows one to feel part of the community of life rather than feeling at odds with it. Yoga taught me, above all, that life provides us with opportunities to be kind. Kindness leads to compassion, and compassion is essential for enlightenment, which is the goal of yoga.

Through the practice of yoga, I have learned something about the nature and meaning of karma. I have come to realize that how we treat others determines our own reality. This reinforced my belief in the reaction Mrs. Goose and I had shared when I was a child—it showed me that I was not, in fact, alone in my view that we are powerful beings whose actions have an impact. What this helped me to see and understand is that this impact is not just on "the world" at large but on everyone around me and, ultimately, on myself. That is what finally motivated me to become a yoga teacher as a way to share the benefits of veganism with others who are interested in the path of enlightenment.

I consider myself an activist—a yoga activist as well as an animal rights activist. What does it mean to be an activist? An activist is someone who actively wants to stimulate a change in the world. We all know that trying to change a situation by pointing fingers and blaming others will only lead to frustration, because it externalizes the problem. It creates a war zone where we are fighting with reality. When you fight with reality, you will always loose. A more positive solution may be found by getting to the root of the issue, which will always lead back to your self. Through deep yogic, contemplative self-inquiry, we can discover how our thoughts, words, and actions create the reality that we live in, and that anger and blame are not valid solutions.

Yoga offers an effective form of activism because it teaches us that there really is no "out there" out there. What we see in the world around us is only a reflection of what is inside of us. Our present reality is a projection of our inner reality, and that inner reality arises according to our past karmas. Our past karmas are the result of how we have treated others. How we have treated others in the past determines our present reality. That's good news.

We create the world we live in. If we want to change what we don't like in the world, we must start by changing what we don't like about ourselves. That is a task we have the power to handle and one that will actually succeed in changing the world.

We are in the midst of a global crisis. Most people (humans, that is) don't realize this. Most people don't realize that *we* are causing the crisis. Many of us who are aware that we are causing this crisis don't know what to do about it. I feel that the popularity of yoga at this time of global crisis is no coincidence. A yogi, by definition, is someone who is striving to live harmoniously with the Earth and, through that good relationship, purify his or her karma so that enlightenment can arise. What is realized in the enlightened state is the oneness of being or the interconnectedness of all beings. Such a shift in consciousness has the potential to elevate our souls out of material and spiritual suffering and save our planet.

INVOCATION

LOKĀḤ SAMASTĀḤ SUKHINO BHAVANTU

May all beings everywhere be happy and free, and may the thoughts, words, and actions of my own life contribute in some way to that happiness and to that freedom for all.

Let's look more closely at this invocational mantra:

lokah: location, realm, all universes existing now
samastah: all beings sharing that same location
sukhino: centered in happiness and joy, free from suffering
bhav: the divine mood or state of unified existence
antu: may it be so, it must be so

(**Antu** used as an ending here transforms this mantra into a powerful pledge.)

This is a prayer each one of us can practice every day. It reminds us that our relationships with all beings and things should be mutually beneficial if we ourselves desire happiness and liberation from suffering. No true or lasting happiness can come from causing unhappiness to others. No true or lasting freedom can come from depriving others of their freedom. If we say we want every being to be happy and free, then we have to question everything that we do—how we live, how we eat, what we buy, how we speak, and even how we think.

Karma means "action." It covers all actions—thought, word, and deed. The law of karma says that for every action there is a reaction. Albert Einstein was reminding us of the law of karma when he pointed out that space is curved. Whatever is thrown out there will eventually but inevitably find its way back to its origin, so we should be careful about what we choose to think, say, or do, because we will be revisited by our actions in due time.

This may be a difficult idea for some of us to grasp, as we have been so thoroughly conditioned by our culture of slavery, violence, and denial. We have been told over and over again that we don't have to take responsibility for our actions and that our individual actions don't matter much to the whole—much less to ourselves. But they do matter; in fact, they are probably the most important and defining aspect of how our future world will be shaped. We ensure our own future suffering by what we do to animals now. These warnings date back thousands of years to the Yoga Sutras, whose dictates are as relevant today as they were then. We each weave our own tangled web of karma and will most certainly become entangled in it, as our reality is being created from our own actions.

The practices of yoga can guide us toward right action and a lifestyle guided by compassionate concern for the happiness of others. The first step toward understanding the link between how we treat others and our own happiness and liberation is to look at the deeper aspects of what the practice of yoga may be able to reveal to us.

INTRODUCTION

I'M A VEGAN BECAUSE TO EAT MEAT AND DAIRY PRODUCTS is a mean thing to do. I don't want to be mean—who wants to be intentionally mean? When we have the choice, isn't it always better to be kind rather than cruel? When people ask me why I don't eat meat or dairy products, I often reply, "I just can't afford it." The expression on their faces is always one of incredulousness. "Oh, come on—I don't believe that," they say, to which I reply, "Well, it's true. Karmically, it is just way too expensive." That usually gives them something to chew on for a while.

My idea is not a new one by any means. It is the same message that Jesus, who embodied all the true qualities of a yogi, gave over two thousand years ago: Treat others as you would like to be treated. Even when Jesus said it, it was old news. Patanjali tried to tell us as much in his Yoga Sutras, written perhaps before Jesus's lifetime. Your present situation—wherever you find yourself, however others are treating you—has been orchestrated long before you were even born. You in your past lives, by your own actions toward others, have sown the seeds for your present reality. The ball's in your court, so to speak. You can change your situation, redirect your destiny, by how you choose to act now and how you choose to relate to others. If you are causing them pain in any way—physical or mental—you will reap the results of those actions in a future time.

That future may be sooner than you think. If you know this, it is actually cause to rejoice, because it means that your situation is in your own hands and is all dependent on how you behave toward others. If you want to be happy, do your very best to make others happy.

Times have changed since 2008, when I wrote the first edition of this book. The once frightening *V*-word (*vegan*) is more acceptable now. Even mainstream TV news anchors pronounce it correctly ("vee-gan" with a long "e" and hard "g"—not "veggen," as they once mistakenly said). Although I was a vegan at the time and had been since 1983, the original title of the first edition was *Yoga and Vegetarianism*. The choice to use *vegetarianism* rather than *veganism* was deliberate. Yes, it made the book more accessible to readers at the time, but more than that, the decision came from my respect for language. I felt strongly about using the word vegetarianism as part of my personal practice of *satya*, truth-telling.

The meaning of words can become corrupted and devolve to such an extent that the current way a word is used can be far removed from its original meaning. The word *vegetarian* originally referred to a person who ate vegetables. Milk is not a vegetable, eggs are not vegetables, fish are not vegetables, and chicken is not a vegetable, nor is honey, and yet it became common for some people who ate these products, which all come from (or are) animals, to call themselves vegetarians. We live in strange times, indeed, and people often do not say what they mean or mean what they say, and so you can't always believe what people tell you. This corruption of the word *vegetarian* became so drastic that a new word was invented to mean "vegetarian." Over the past few years, the word *vegan* has come to mean (in English as well as other languages) "a person who eats a plant-based diet, as well as one who extends his or her concept of consumption to exclude all products derived from animal sources."

Just in the last decade, there has been a shift in consciousness and a wider acceptance of veganism for health, environmental, animal rights, and spiritual reasons. Many medical doctors are challenging the established standard American diet (SAD) of meat, dairy, and processed foods promoted by the advertising agencies and lobbyists who are employed by the animal-user industries and, instead, suggesting healthy plant-based alternatives. More and more environmentalists are seeing the connection between the devastation of our planet's ecosystem and raising animals to feed the growing human population.

Due to the courageous work of many animal rights activists who fearlessly speak up and show the world the horrid suffering of animals locked behind closed doors in laboratories and factory farms, the mainstream public can no longer cite ignorance to justify bad behavior. Seeing and hearing the truth—revealed through films, books, blogs, etc.—has awakened many, and the human heart's capacity for extending compassion to include other animals has grown, making this world a kinder place for all inhabitants.

Due to the enlightened efforts of many people, the important connection between spiritual practice and our actions in the world—for example, how we treat others and the planet and how that interaction affects ourselves and the world, physically as well as spiritually—has become more clear. With that clarity, the urgency of the problem has begun to appear along with a call to spiritual activism. The most important thing that any of us can do is to dare to care about the happiness and well-being of others.

The concept of ahimsa, or not causing harm to another, has been around for centuries. It is introduced in the foundational teachings of Yoga, Buddhism, and all major spiritual traditions and religions in the world. But it has mostly been applied only to other human beings—and limited further to exclude people who you don't like so well. Extending the concept of ahimsa to include animals and extending the practice of ahimsa to not eating animals or exploiting them in any way are two very new ideas.

Although I do cite health, environmental concerns, and animal rights as reasons to go vegan, the premise of this book is to provide a logical argument in favor of veganism from the viewpoint of classical yoga philosophy, in particular drawing from four concepts found in the second chapter (the chapter on practice) of Patanjali's Yoga Sutras: kriya yoga (PYS II.1), the five kleshas (PYS II.3), the yamas (PYS II.29), and asana (PYS II.46).

When many people think of yoga, they think of ahimsa, or nonviolence. Yes, ahimsa is a no-brainer when it comes to a reason to make the vegan choice, but it is only one of the five yamas. I invite you to come with me as we venture even further than ahimsa to find a strong, commonsense, conclusive, solid case for veganism in the Yoga Sutras, and together we can activate a spiritual revolution that will bring about an enlightened transformation in the way we see and relate to others, the world, and ourselves.

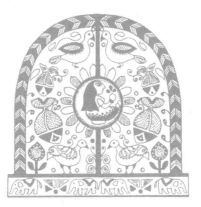

CHAPTER I

WHAT DOES YOGA HAVE TO DO WITH VEGANISM?

Questioning Old Habits

The most important part of the yoga practice is . . . diet.
—SRI K. PATTABHI JOIS

THE SANSKRIT TERM *YOGA* IS FOUND IN THE VEDAS, THE most ancient of the Indian scriptures, prehistoric in origin. The Indian philosopher Patanjali did not invent yoga, but he did write an important manual, the Yoga Sutras. The word *yoga* is derived from the Sanskrit *yuj*, which means "to yoke," and describes the yoking of one's individual small self to the cosmic eternal Self, or God. Reaching this blissful state of union with the Divine is called enlightenment, liberation, Self-realization, superconsciousness, or *samadhi*. Jesus referred to this state when he reputedly said, "I and my father are one." In all probability, he didn't use the English word *father*. Most likely, he used *Alaha*, the Aramaic term for the Divine, which means "the interconnectedness of all beings and things: the oneness of being." A more apt biblical translation of that New Testament passage might be, "I know myself as one with all that is." Jesus was describing Yogic enlightenment. When this enlightenment happens, the presence of God enraptures the soul, freeing it from the tyrannical dictates of the ego and its insatiable desire to lord over others and the Earth. The person exudes from their entire being this emancipation. They are known as a *jivanmukta*, one who is living liberated.

When Patanjali states, "*Yogah chitta-vritti-nirodhah*" in the first chapter of the Yoga Sutras, he is giving us both a definition of Yoga and a directive as to how to attain it. This sutra can be translated as "When you stop (*nirodhah*) identifying with the divisive nature of your mind (*chitta vritti*), then there is Yoga (*yogah*), which is enlightenment." The union of the separate with the whole implies that enlightenment is actually the underlying ground of being and that otherness is an imposition or distortion of a more unified reality.

If we are interested in Yoga, we might ask ourselves, "What is Yoga interested in?" Yoga has one goal: enlightenment, a state in which the separateness of self and other dissolves in the realization of the oneness of being. What holds us back from that realization is a false perception of reality. Instead of perceiving oneness, we see separateness, disconnection, and otherness. Because the term *Yoga* refers not only to the goal of enlightenment but also to the practical method for reaching that goal, all of the practices must address the basic issue of "other." Otherness is the main obstacle to enlightenment. Killing or harming others is not the best way to overcome that obstacle. How we perceive and relate to the others in our lives determines whether enlightenment arises.

When most people think of yoga, they think of the physical postures taught in yoga classes. This is a yoga practice called *asana*, but the true meaning of the term beyond physical fitness is not well understood. Most practitioners even think of asana practice as a form of gymlike exercise undertaken to increase strength and flexibility and perhaps reduce stress. Some may understand it as one of the many yoga practices, such as meditation, *pranayama* (directing the life force through breathing exercises), and yama (restraining your behavior toward others), that can help us realize our true nature. But still they may not see the practice of asana as a way to perfect one's relationship to the Earth and all beings.

What is a perfect relationship? One that is not one-sided or selfish but mutually beneficial. If we are still eating meat, fish, or dairy products, we might question whether our relationship to the animals we are eating is mutually beneficial and, with that answer, decide if our eating choices serve our ultimate goal: the attainment of Yoga. When yoga practitioners understand the fuller meaning of asana as relationship with the Earth, their practice takes on a deeper dimension and becomes spiritual activism.

Compassion brings about the arising of enlightenment. But what is compassion? Is it the same as empathy or sympathy? No. *Sympathy* is to recognize that someone is in pain, *empathy* is not only to recognize the pain of the other but to feel it as if it is happening to you. Compassion, however, raises the bar a few notches. A compassionate person recognizes that someone else is in pain and feels that pain but is committed to figuring out how to alleviate it. *Compassion* literally means "feel together," but the term also encompasses the motivation to relieve the suffering, understanding that when you relieve the suffering of another, your own suffering will be gone, too. All yoga practices are designed to help one develop compassion and, by means of compassion, dissolve the illusion of otherness. Through the practice of compassion, you begin to realize that everyone else in your life is really coming from inside you. Through compassion, you are able to not only acknowledge this but also absorb everyone back into the fullness (or emptiness) of your own being. In Yogic terminology, this is referred to as *shunyata*, or emptiness (or fullness, if you want to see it that way).

Our experience of everything we see and everyone we meet is colored by our own perceptions. We are actually the most important people in our lives because we determine who the others are and what significance they hold. This is not a subjective occurrence that happens consciously in the moment of perception, but rather a conditioned response developed over time through repeated actions or karmas. These karmas plant the seeds that create our understanding of others, of reality, and of ourselves.

Yoga teaches us that we can have whatever we may want in life if we are willing to provide it for others first. In fact, whatever we are experiencing in our lives is a direct result of how we have treated others in our past. The way we treat others will determine how others treat us. After all, they are only acting as agents of our own karmas. How others treat us will influence how we see ourselves. How we see ourselves will greatly determine who we are, and who we are will be revealed in our actions.

The others in our world can provide us with the opportunities we need to evolve. The world will either keep us in bondage or provide us with the means to liberation. When we give to others that which we want for ourselves—when an action is selfless—it leads to the type of karma that will eventually lead to liberation.

As yogis seeking liberation, we strive to perfect our actions. Every action is preceded by a thought. To perfect an action, we must therefore first perfect our thoughts. What is a perfect thought? A perfect thought is one devoid of selfish motive: free of anger, greed, hate, jealousy, and the like.

If you wish to truly step into transcendental reality and have a lighter impact on the planet, adopting a compassionate vegan diet is a good place to start. Not everyone can stand on his or her head every day, but everyone eats. You can practice compassion three times a day when you sit down to eat. This is one of the many reasons that so many yoga practitioners choose to be vegans.

Ethical vegetarians eat only plant-based food in order to show compassion toward animals and other humans and to benefit the planet. Some people say they are vegetarian but still eat milk products, eggs, and fish. Ethical vegetarians do not eat dairy products, eggs, and fish because these are not vegetables and eating them causes great harm to other beings and the planet. Vegans are ethical vegetarians who seek to extend their ethics to include not just what they eat but everything they consume: food, clothing, medicine, fuel, and entertainment, to name a few.

The term *veganism* was coined in 1944 by Donald Watson (1910–2005), who founded the Vegan Society in England. Vegans do their best to refrain from exploiting animals for any reason and believe that animals do not exist as slaves to serve human beings. A vegan is a strict ethical vegetarian who abstains from eating or using any products that have been derived from animal sources. The mission statement of PETA sums it up this way: "Animals are not ours to use for food, clothing, laboratory experimentation, entertainment, or any other exploitative purpose."

Some meat eaters defend their choice by saying that it is natural, because animals eat one another in the wild. When people bring this up as a rationale for eating meat, I remind them that the animals that end up on our plates aren't those who eat one another in the wild. The animals we regularly exploit for food are not the lions, tigers, and bears of the world. Our preference is to eat the gentle ones like cows and lambs—vegan animals who, if given the choice, would never eat the flesh of other animals, although they are forced to do so on today's farms when they are fed "enriched feed" containing rendered animal parts.3

---

3 Joe Loria, "What They Feed Animals on Factory Farms Is Disgusting," Mercy for Animals (March 2, 2017), http://www.mercyforanimals.org/what-they-feed-animals-on-factory-farms-is.

Some may say a vegan diet is difficult to follow. What does *difficult* mean? How difficult is it to suffer and die from heart disease caused by a diet high in saturated fats and cholesterol? Still, many people would choose to go through invasive bypass surgery or have a breast, colon, or rectum removed and take powerful pharmaceutical drugs for the rest of their lives rather than change their diets because they think veganism is drastic and extreme. How difficult is it for the beings who suffer degrading confinement and cruel slaughter, dying for our dining convenience? How difficult is it for all of us to be confronted with the effects of global warming, deforestation, species extinction, and water, soil, and air pollution, which are a direct result of raising confined animals for food?

How difficult is it for us to endure being hurt and abused, being lied to, worrying about money and security, experiencing mental and physical illnesses, and not knowing what is in store for us next? The five yamas found in Patanjali's Yoga Sutras explain how to curb our behavior toward others in order to alleviate suffering in our own lives. The Sanskrit term *yama* means "to restrict." In the context of the Yoga Sutras, Patanjali provides direct correlations between how we treat others and what we experience. For example, if we don't want to be hurt, we should not hurt others (*ahimsa*); if we don't want to be lied to, we should not lie (*satya*); if we don't want to live in poverty, we should not steal (*asteya*); if we want to enjoy good health, we should not abuse others sexually (*brahmacharya*); if we want to know the purpose of our lives, we should curb our tendency to be greedy (*aparigraha*). The five yamas reveal the karmic effects we can expect to experience when we exploit, kill, and eat animals, which involve harming, deceit, stealing, sexual abuse, and greed. By following the yamas prescribed in Patanjali's Yoga Sutras, we begin to realize that suffering is optional for those who are enlightened about the truth—the interconnectedness between us all and how karma works.

Many are beginning to recognize that planet Earth is in the midst of an ecological crisis. But not many understand that the cause that underlies the global crisis in the world today is a spiritual one. As a species, we human beings do not realize how interconnected we truly are with all of the inhabitants of the world. Most of us are ignorant of the part we play and how our individual actions affect the lives of others, the planet, and even ourselves. Our own actions, collectively as well as individually, have brought about the situation we live in. Yoga has the potential to heal the disease we are all suffering from—the disease of disconnection, which is brought on by ignorance, known in yogic terminology as *avidya*. Avidya is one of the kleshas, or obstacles to enlightenment—it means being ignorant of your true Divine nature and the ways you are interdependent with all of life. War, destruction of the environment, extinction of species, global warming, and even domestic violence—all of these stem from the disease of disconnection. You can abuse and exploit others only if you feel disconnected from them and have no idea of the potency inherent in your own actions. If you feel connected, you know that it's *you*, as well as other living beings and things, who will suffer from the suffering you inflict.

It is wise for the yogi to consider that killing and eating another being perpetuates the wheel of *samsara*—commonly known as the cycle of birth, life, and death. The literal translation of the Sanskrit term *samsara* is "same agitation"—or, one could say, repeating the same mistakes that continue to cause one to experience suffering again and again, life after life. Yoga practitioners are attempting to be free of samsara and, therefore, would want to step out of the so-called natural cycle of the dog-eat-dog world. This would motivate them to consider their actions carefully.

Some may argue that human beings have been doing certain activities "forever" and that, therefore, they are normal and natural and that people should be allowed to continue to do them. However, the fact that a belief or behavior is long held does not make it inherently just, or even right. Consider, for example, the tragic fact that rape has been committed for countless years throughout human history. Does this mean that such behavior is normal and should be allowed to continue?

We are fortunate enough to live in an era in which human beings have come to recognize rape as a crime, at least in the realm of human interaction. We have yet to see the rape of an animal by a human being as a crime, and yet it is what happens to millions of confined animals in the animal agribusiness of the world today. It is often referred to as artificial insemination, but nonetheless, it is rape—forced sexual abuse inflicted on defenseless animals without their consent. (See chapter 6, "Brahmacharya: Good Sex.")

We have a double standard in our culture that sanctions certain behavior, like theft, rape, and murder, when it is perpetrated on others who have been deemed as unworthy of our respect. As children, we are taught that prejudice against others in the name of patriarchy, nationalism, economics, war, or species is okay. For example, during wartime, when nations view each other as the enemy, killing is not only an accepted behavior but is also taught and promoted. Throughout history, when a victorious army conquers a town, the soldiers are encouraged to take the spoils of war, which often include the right to pillage and rape. This still occurs in our society today. Similarly, it could be said that we are at war with animals. As a culture, we do not see animals as we see ourselves—as people, living beings deserving of respect; we see them as inferior, less than, the "other."

During war, a lot of energy is devoted to propaganda—promoting hate and prejudice against the other. The habitual exploitation and killing of animals has long been the central foundation of our global economy, and with it has come the development and maintenance of the deep-rooted psychology of speciesism—the prejudice against nonhuman animals.

Prejudices can motivate people to behave callously and feel authorized to perform hideous actions. The fact that we are loathe to admit is that for thousands of years, we have been blinded by our prejudice toward animals and have not been able to see them as the people they are.4 Speciesism has clouded our better judgment, disconnected us from our soul's innate compassion, and allowed us to enslave and degrade

---

4   People for the Ethical Treatment of Animals (PETA), "Joaquin Phoenix Reminds Us That 'We Are All Animals,'" PETA, http://www.peta.org/features/joaquin-phoenix-we-are-all-animals-end-speciesism.

other animals, inflicting horrendous pain and suffering on them. The sheer numbers of animals tortured and slaughtered every minute all over the globe is at an all-time high, and because of that, we are experiencing the backlash of our actions in an unprecedented way. It is time that we consider what we are doing.

A yogi investigates *all* long-standing habits and behaviors, even if they have been in place seemingly forever, and asks, "Is this activity necessary now? Does it prolong or diminish suffering and bring me or the world closer to enlightenment or peace?"

Besides the yamas, from another point of view, a yogi might consider the *kleshas* as a reason for veganism. *Klesha* means "obstruction." Patanjali discloses that there are five main obstacles to the attainment of a concentrated, clear, calm, serene mind—a necessary ingredient for yoga and freedom from samsara. The kleshas are introduced in the beginning of the second chapter of the Yoga Sutras, even before the mention of the yamas.

avidyā-asmitā-rāga-dveṣa-abhiniveśāḥ pañca kleśāḥ
PYS II.3

The five kleshas are *avidya* (ignorance of your Divine nature), *asmita* (identification with ego and the material body), *raga* (attachment to what you like), *dvesha* (hate or aversion to what you don't like), and *abhinivesha* (fear of death). The kleshas are afflictions, pain-bearing obstacles that at their core are the result of an ignorant misperception of yourself and others, and with that a forgetfulness of your connection to God and the goodness of your eternal soul. These obstructions contribute to our selfishness, prejudices, preferences, fearfulness, and stupid and destructive habits.

Eating meat is a long-standing habit in our culture. Even some Western yoga practitioners argue that they have to eat meat to keep up the strength required for a physically demanding asana practice. Yet Sri K. Pattabhi Jois, the Indian master of the physically demanding style of Ashtanga yoga, has stated clearly that a vegetarian diet is a requirement for the practice of yoga. He was initially very reluctant to teach Western students because they were meat eaters, and it was only in the last twenty years or so that he has opened his doors wide to Western students. I had assumed the reason was that he felt there would be language difficulties, but when I asked him to confirm, he replied, "No. It was because they weren't vegetarians. If someone is not a vegetarian, they won't be able to learn yoga. They will be too stiff in their body and their mind."

"But, Guruji," I said, "you teach mostly Western students now. What caused you to change?"

"In my country, we are vegetarians because our parents are; we were born that way," he replied. "At first, when Westerners came to me, I assumed a lot about them. Most Indian people do. But then some students came to me, and I learned that they were vegetarians, and they weren't born that way. They had decided on their own to become vegetarians. This seemed very unusual, and I felt that it was interesting and significant. And so I began teaching them because I felt they could learn."

The popularity of yoga worldwide has grown tremendously in the midst of a global crisis. This is no coincidence. Yoga holds the promise that could help us transform our ways of relating to animals, the Earth, and one another. Through yoga practice, we purify our past karmas and in turn develop Self-confidence. We begin to feel like integrated beings as we start to heal the disease of disconnection that has separated our hearts from our minds and our bodies. Then the illusion that we are separate from the rest of creation begins to dissolve. With that disconnection dissolved, we begin to perceive our connection to the Divine, and the truth of who we really are is revealed. And with that revelation, we behave differently toward the Earth; we become more other-centered. We see from the expanded perspective of "we" rather than "me."

I am thankful that yoga is being embraced in our Western culture by a growing minority, because we desperately need to stop viewing the Earth and all other beings as ours to exploit. Much of our culture's influence has been negative and quite destructive, based on the lie that "the Earth belongs to us." Yoga has always opposed this proprietary worldview and has offered humanity an alternative over the centuries: the means to live harmoniously with the Earth and all beings. If human beings can't find a new way to live *with* this planet, our own annihilation, as well as the planet's, is certain. Without planetary harmony, no cosmic harmony can be hoped for. I believe that the teachings and practices of yoga are very important, perhaps even crucial, for the survival of life on Earth.

That is why I am passionate about practicing and teaching yoga.

The choice to become yogis and the choices we make about what to eat are karmic, political, and economic decisions that affect our mental and physical health. They have repercussions in our families as well as in our larger communities. It is an indisputable fact that a vegan diet causes less harm to ourselves, to animals, to plants, and to the Earth. To say that what you choose to eat is nobody else's business is to belittle yourself and deny the impact that your actions have upon the lives of others.

There are many reasons a person might choose to be vegan. For a normal person, they are health, the environment, and animal rights. It is a proven scientific medical fact that eating a vegan diet is better for human *health*. There is strong evidence linking the leading diseases of our time—heart disease, cancer, and diabetes—to eating a meat- and dairy-based diet, and there are an overwhelming number of proven cases of the reversal of those diseases in patients after they adopt a vegan diet.[5]

From an *environmental* point of view, eating a plant-based diet is better for the planet. There are many findings to support this. The livestock industry is the single biggest contributor to global warming, as it creates far more greenhouse gas emissions than all forms of transportation

---

5 C. B. Esselstyn Jr., MD, FACS, http://www.dresselstyn.com; Dean Ornish, MD, http://www.ornish.com/proven-program/nutrition; and Neal Bernard, MD, http://www.pcrm.org/health-topics/cancer and http://www.pcrm.org/health-topics/diabetes. See also http://www.gamechangersmovie.com/benefits/optimizing-health.

combined!6 There are more cows (most of them hidden from our view) in the United States than there are human beings. The biggest consumers of fresh water are the meat and dairy industries. They are also responsible for most of the water pollution and for the increase of dangerous toxic chemicals found in our water, soil, and air, as well as in our bodies. Most of the plant food—soybeans, corn, oats, and so on—that are grown to be fed to livestock are saturated with toxic chemicals, pesticides, and herbicides and are genetically modified. The development of food derived from genetically modified organisms (GMOs) to feed to livestock is on the rise.

So, plants fed to livestock are not healthy, which in turn compromises the health of the animals, who are given antibiotics and other pharmaceutical drugs to keep them alive long enough to go to slaughter, and human beings then eat those unhealthy animals. The residue from the chemicals in the plants, as well as the drugs fed to confined animals, end up not only in the flesh, blood, and milk of those animals but also in their excrement, which goes down the drains and into our water systems to eventually but inevitably contaminate our drinking water. These are just a few ways that the meat and dairy industries are devastating our environment.

From an *animal rights* perspective, veganism is the kinder choice; enslaving and abusing animals is cruel. The mass murder of billions of gentle beings every minute of every day is business as usual in our world. By subjecting animals to lifelong torture and degradation, we

---

6 Food and Agriculture Organization of the United Nations (FAO), *Livestock's Long Shadow: Environmental Issues and Options* (FAO, 2006).

deprive them of their rights to freedom and happiness. How can we ourselves hope to be free or happy when our own lives are rooted in depriving others of the very thing we say we value most in life—the freedom to pursue happiness? If you want to bring more peace and happiness into your own life, the way to do so is to stop causing violence and unhappiness in the lives of others.

Health, environmental concerns, and animal rights are all great reasons to go vegan, but there are also other reasons that could compel a yogi, in particular, to choose veganism, and it is those reasons that I will explore more fully in this book.

Yoga reminds us that all of life is sacred, that all of life is connected, and that what we do to another, we eventually do to ourselves. The best way to uplift our own lives is to do all we can to uplift the lives of others.

How we behave toward others and our environment reveals—more than anything else—our inner state of mind and the current condition of our personalities. How have we become so estranged from our true Divine nature and from nature herself? Are human beings naturally violent, deceitful, selfish, manipulative, and greedy? Or have we learned and perfected these negative traits over time? Could the practice of yoga not only challenge the basic assumptions expressed by these negative traits but also reverse them and, in doing so, allow us to recreate ourselves, our societies, and the world we live in?

In the beginning of the second chapter of the Yoga Sutras, Patanjali outlines for us the main obstructions to yoga as the five kleshas; later, he lays out an eight-limbed plan for liberation called Raja yoga. The first limb is called *yama* (restraint), and it includes five ethical restrictions.

---

ahiṁsā-satyāsteya-brahmacharyāparigrahā yamāḥ
PYS II.30

---

1. **ahimsa:** nonharming
2. **satya:** truthfulness
3. **asteya:** nonstealing
4. **brahmacharya:** sexual continence
5. **aparigraha:** greedlessness

The yamas describe how an unenlightened person who desires Yoga should restrict his or her behavior toward others. Patanjali says that as long as you still perceive "others" and not one interconnected reality, then 1) don't harm others, 2) don't deceive them, 3) don't steal from them, 4) don't manipulate them sexually, and 5) don't be greedy, selfishly depriving them of sustenance and happiness. Through the practice of yama, Patanjali tells us that we can begin to purify our karmas and remove the obstacles to our enlightenment, which are rooted in our misperception of others.

In this book, we investigate how the yamas relate to veganism, as well as what one can expect as a result of being established in the practice of each of the yamas. This is called *pratishthayam*, which means "become established in." Patanjali suggests that if we work for the freedom of other beings, we will become free. By becoming established in the practice of the yamas, we can look forward to a peaceful world free of violence (through *ahimsa*), lies (through *satya*), and stealing (through *asteya*); the enjoyment of physical and mental vitality and the end of disease (through *brahmacharya*); and a future free of poverty and bright with opportunities for increased happiness and creativity (through *aparigraha*).

What would we find if we were to investigate the yamas in terms of how we are treating the animals we put on our plates every day? Are we harming them? Are we deceiving them? Are we stealing from them? Are we manipulating them sexually? Are we impoverishing them through our greed? What impact does our treatment of these "other" animals have on our inner and outer environment?

Don't wait for a better world. Start now to create a world of harmony and peace. It is up to you, and it always has been! You may even find the solution at the end of your fork.

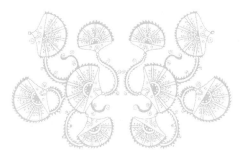

CHAPTER 2

ASANA

Our Connection to the Earth and All Beings

*We have come into this world to bring peace and
happiness to all beings. To achieve this goal, it is
necessary to adopt peaceful ways of harmless living
and noninterference in the happiness of others.*

—SWAMI NIRMALANANDA

*We have been at war with the other creatures of this
Earth ever since the first human hunter set forth with
spear into the primeval forest. Human imperialism has
everywhere enslaved, oppressed, murdered, and mutilated
the animal peoples. All around us lie the slave camps
we have built for our fellow creatures, factory farms
and vivisection laboratories, Dachaus and Buchenwalds
for the conquered species. We slaughter animals for our
food, force them to perform silly tricks for our delection,
gun them down and stick hooks in them in the name of
sport. We have torn up the wild places where once they
made their homes. Speciesism is more deeply entrenched
within us than sexism, and that is deep enough.*

—RON LEE, FOUNDER OF THE ANIMAL LIBERATION FRONT

sthira-sukham āsanam PYS II.46
The connection to the Earth should be steady and joyful.

sthira: steady
sukham: joyful
asanam: seat (connection to the Earth)

WHEN MOST PEOPLE THINK OF YOGA, THEY THINK OF the physical postures called *asana*. In fact, Patanjali mentions asana only twice in the Yoga Sutras, but when he does he provides us with a powerful means to purify our relationships with others.

There is a misperception that asana is done in preparation for the "higher" yogic practices, such as meditation. This is not true. In the Yoga Sutras, Patanjali gives asana equal importance to meditation as a practice for reaching awareness of the oneness of all being. *Sthira* means "steady," and *sukham* means "joyful and comfortable." In our contemporary times, *asana* is usually translated as "pose" or "posture." The original meaning of the Sanskrit word is "seat." (The English word *ass* is cognate with *asana*.) Patanjali is addressing those who seek enlightenment. He tells them that, in order to achieve enlightenment, their connection (or relationship) to the Earth—which refers to all beings and things—must be both steady and joyful. Currently, our connection to the Earth is dangerously out of balance, and asana practice can provide much-needed insight into how to improve it.

Asana practice is beneficial on many levels. It has been shown to help restore flexibility and strength, to be therapeutic for injuries, and to balance hormonal secretions, supporting youthfulness. For one who desires enlightenment, asana practice is especially valuable because it provides an opportunity to purify one's karmas. Because our bodies are storehouses for all of our past karmas, and our physical bodies are made from the food that we eat, imbalances show up as tightness, uptightness, discomfort, and even disease. Through the deeply therapeutic practice of asana, we begin to purify our karmas, thereby healing our past relationships with others and reestablishing a steady and joyful connection with the Earth, which means all of life.

With *sthira-sukham asanam*, Patanjali is proposing a radical idea that, if realized and put into practice, could stop the war that human beings have been waging against animals and Mother Nature for the past 10,000 years. With the conclusion of that war, we could begin to build a new world and a harmonious and sustainable way of living based on joy and mutual benefit.

Is there a contradiction between spirituality and veganism, environmentalism, or animal rights activism? The latter three are associated with politics, and many yogis have been cautioned not to mix spirituality with politics. But let's look deeper into what the word *politic* really means. *Politic* means "body." The word can also mean "the greater body," implying the extended body or community. Being political means "to care about the politic"—the community of others we live with. The term *dharma* literally means "to hold together," which is what a body does. In this sense, being politically active has a dharmic connotation. To choose to be aware of how one's actions may affect others is to become politically active. To care about other beings and act on their behalf is therefore very much in line with the teachings of yoga.

If we, as a species, are ever going to find a way to live peacefully—which implies fearlessly—then we must look to our relationship with creation itself to see where the obstacles to peace arise. The practice of asana allows us to investigate our physiology and psychology. If we have been eating meat and dairy products, we have bodies that are not only filled with toxins hazardous to our health (in the form of pesticides, herbicides, and antibiotics and other pharmaceutical drugs) but also composed of the karmic results of violence, cruelty, fear, terror, and despair. Through asana practice, we begin to notice how our diet may be contributing to tightness and constriction in our bodies and minds and an uneasy feeling of imbalance with ourselves and others.

We may also notice, as we go deeper into our asana practice, that the prevalent disease in our culture is low self-esteem. Perhaps we feel bad about ourselves if we can't execute a yoga asana perfectly. As we watch our thoughts spin into a downward spiral, we may begin to realize that our culture has done an excellent job of making us all feel fearful and quite inadequate. This lack of self-confidence may cause us to think that what we do as an individual doesn't matter much to the whole and that our actions are insignificant. If we feel this way, we may not believe that we are responsible for our own lives and that we have a profound effect on the lives of others and the world around us. We may even feel unworthy of spiritual attainment and think that enlightenment is reserved only for people like Ramakrishna, Buddha, or Mother Teresa. The practice of yoga has the power to shatter and dissolve these misconceptions, but it might take a lot of transformational work to accomplish that.

Ours is not a meditative, self-reflecting culture. We are a distracted, gotta-get-up-and-do-something culture, always seeking stimulation from the outside. For a meat eater to be calm enough to come to a yoga mat or meditation cushion and surrender to deep contemplation can be quite difficult, perhaps because it will be hard to bear the truth of what might be found inside: the shadow that has been denied. From its inception, our culture has participated in the brutal reality of the enslavement and eating of animals. If we eat meat, we carry in our bodies the karmic repercussions of the pain we have inflicted on these animals we are consuming. Even if we are vegans and don't eat animals, we still live in an atmosphere where this is happening, and on some level, we feel the suffering.

Through the benefits that arise from practicing yoga, and not just from reading or hearing about it, we may discover that cultivating kindness improves our sense of well-being, our peace of mind, and our physical health. On the other hand, violence and selfish habits lead ultimately to physical, mental, spiritual, and environmental breakdown.

"Most people's relationship to animals occurs three times a day when they sit down to eat them—that's a terrible way to define a relationship!" says activist Ingrid Newkirk. Contrary to popular belief, the animal nations do not belong to us, and we will ultimately not benefit by exploiting them for our shortsighted gain. The yogi strives to live in harmony with Mother Nature and, through her blessings, attain enlightenment—the knowledge of the absolute reality. This is the underlying reason that eating a vegan diet, which minimizes one's exploitation of animals and the environment, is of vital importance. Eating a vegan diet can contribute more to saving ourselves and the planet than any other single effort.

Our meat-eating culture not only affects the animals that are tortured and killed but also causes tremendous worldwide environmental devastation— which scientists loudly proclaim will have catastrophic effects on the planet.

Some facts:

1. Global warming: According to the United Nations, raising animals for food creates more greenhouse gas emissions than all the transportation (cars, trucks, buses, trains, planes, ships, etc.) in the world.[7] This is the *real* "inconvenient truth." A person who follows a vegan diet produces the equivalent of 50 percent less carbon dioxide and uses one-eleventh the oil a meat-eater uses.[8]

---

7 FAO, *Livestock's Long Shadow*; PETA, "Fight Climate Change by Going Vegan," PETA, http://www.peta.org/issues/animals-used-for-food/global-warming.

8 Janet Ranganathan and Richard Waite, "Sustainable Diets: What You Need to Know in 12 Charts." World Resources Institute (April 2016), https://www.wri.org/blog/2016/04/sustainable-diets-what-you-need-know-12-charts.

2. Water pollution: In the United States, raising animals for food causes more water pollution than any other industry.[9] These animals produce 130 times the waste of the entire human population of the United States, 87,000 pounds of waste per second.[10] A farm with 2,500 dairy cows produces the same amount of waste as a city of 411,000 people.[11] Much of the waste from factory farms—which contains high levels of toxic chemicals from pesticides, herbicides, and antibiotics, hormones, and other pharmaceuticals—flows into and contaminates streams, rivers, and oceans as well as our drinking water.[12]

3. Water use: More than half the water consumed in the United States is used to raise animals for food.[13] It takes 2,500 gallons of water to produce

9 Frances Moore Lappé, *Diet for a Small Planet* (New York: Ballantine, 1971), 22. See also Richard Oppenlander, "Freshwater Abuse and Loss: Where Is It All Going?," Forks Over Knives, May 20, 2013, https://www.forksoverknives.com/freshwater-abuse-and-loss-where-is-it-all-going/#gs.8e3f1g.

10 Ed Ayres, "Will We Still Eat Meat?," *Time* November 8, 1999, http://content.time.com/time/magazine/article/0,9171,992523,00.html. See also the U.S. Senate Committee on Agriculture's 1997 report "Animal Waste Pollution in America: An Emerging National Problem" and U.S. General Accounting Office (GAO), "Animal Agriculture: Waste Management Practices," GAO (1999), https://www.gao.gov/archive/1999/rc99205.pdf.

11 U.S. Environmental Protection Agency (EPA), "Risk Assessment Evaluation for Concentrated Animal Feeding Operations," EPA, 2004 See also FAO, http://www.fao.org/home/en.

12 FAO, "More People, More Food, Worse Water? A Global Review of Water Pollution from Agriculture," FAO and the International Water Management Institute, 2018, http://www.fao.org/3/ca0146en/CA0146EN.pdf.

13 Frances Moore Lappé, *Diet for a Small Planet*, 10th ed. (New York: Ballantine, 1982), 69. See also https://www.cowspiracy.com/facts.

1 pound of beef,[14] but only 25 gallons to produce 1 pound of wheat.[15] It takes 477 gallons of water to produce 1 pound of eggs; almost 900 gallons of water are needed for 1 pound of cheese.[16] It takes an entire months' worth of showers to produce just 1 gallon of milk, and an estimated 4,200 gallons of water per day to produce the average meat-and-dairy diet. The production of an average plant-based diet, by comparison, requires 300 gallons of water per day.[17]

4. Oceans: The world's oceans are being emptied of life; we could see fishless oceans by 2048.[18] Each year, 90–100 million tons of fish are pulled from our oceans.[19] As many as 2.7 trillion additional animals are pulled from the ocean each year.[20] For every 1 pound of fish caught, up to 5 pounds of unintended marine species are caught and discarded as by-kill.[21] As many as 40

14 Matt Moore, "Institute Warns of Possible Water Shortage," Associated Press, April 20, 2004. See also Water Footprint Network, "Water Footprint of Crop and Animal Products: A Comparison," Water Footprint Network, https://waterfootprint.org/en/water-footprint/product-water-footprint/water-footprint-crop-and-animal-products.

15 Robbins, The Food Revolution, 236.

16 Water Education Foundation, "Food Facts: How Much Water Does it Take to Produce . . . ?," Water Education Foundation, https://www.watereducation.org/post/food-facts-how-much-water-does-it-take-produce.

17 Aisling Maria Cronin, "You Can Save Over 200,000 Gallons of Water a Year with One Simple Choice," One Green Planet, https://www.onegreenplanet.org/environment/how-to-save-water-with-one-simple-choice.

18 John Roach, "Seafood May Be Gone by 2048, Study Says," National Geographic, November 2, 2006, https://www.nationalgeographic.com/animals/2006/11/seafood-biodiversity.

19 FAO, "World Review of Fisheries and Aquaculture: Part 1," FAO, http://www.fao.org/3/i2727e/i2727e01.pdf.

20 A. Mood and P. Brooke, "Estimating the Number of Fish Caught in Global Fishing Each Year," Fishcount.org.uk, http://www.fishcount.org.uk/published/std/fishcountstudy.pdf.

21 FAO, "Discard and Bycatch in Shrimp Trawl Fisheries," FAO, http://www.fao.org/3/W6602E/w6602E09.htm.

percent of fish caught globally every year (63 billion pounds) are discarded simply because they were not the type of fish the fishermen were fishing for.[22] Scientists estimate that as many as 650,000 whales, dolphins, and seals are killed every year by fishing vessels.[23] Most of the fish and other sea creatures caught annually are not eaten directly by humans but are fed to livestock. It may take 12 pounds of grain to make 1 pound of beef, but it also takes 100 pounds of fish to produce that pound of beef. It takes 50 pounds of wild fish to feed one factory farm–raised salmon.[24]

5. Land: Of all the agricultural land in the United States, 80 percent is used to raise animals for food and the crops to feed them.[25] That's 45 percent of the total 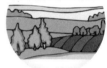 landmass in the United States. According to the United Nations, global land use for farms could be reduced by more than 75 percent— an area equivalent to the United States, China, the European Union, and Australia combined—and still feed the entire world if everyone went vegan.[26] A 2019 climate change report from the United Nations says,

22 Amanda Keledjian et al., "Wasted Catch: Unsolved Problems in U.S. Fisheries," *Oceana* (March 2014), http://oceana.org/sites/default/files/reports/Bycatch_Report_FINAL.pdf.

23 Suzanne Goldenberg, "America's Nine Most Wasteful Fisheries Named," *Guardian*, March 20, 2014, https://www.theguardian.com/environment/2014/mar/20/americas-nine-most-wasteful-fisheries-named.

24 Paul Watson, "Consider the Fishes," *VegNews* (March–April 2003): 27.

25 Kenneth S. Krupa and Marlowe Vesterby. "Major Uses of Land in the United States," *Statistical Bulletin No. 973*, U.S. Department of Agriculture (USDA), 1997. See also "Irrigation and Water Use," USDA, https://www.ers.usda.gov/topics/farm-practices-management/irrigation-water-use/background.aspx.

26 Intergovernmental Panel on Climate Change (IPCC), "Report on the Ocean and Cryosphere in a Changing Climate," IPCC, 2019, https://www.ipcc.ch/srocc/home.

"This sort of change won't come from any industry or government body—it will happen only when we all stop eating animals."

Land required to feed 1 person for 1 year:

VEGAN: $\frac{1}{6}$th acre
VEGETARIAN: 3 times as much as a vegan
MEAT EATER: 18 times as much as a vegan[27]

6. Deforestation: Our wild forests, which are habitats for wild animals, are disappearing. It is estimated that up to 137 plant, animal, and insect species are lost every day due to animal agriculture and its resultant deforestation.[28] One-third of the planet is desertified, with livestock as the leading driver.[29] Animal agriculture is responsible for up to 91 percent of Amazon rain forest destruction.[30] An acre of land disappears every eight seconds worldwide, cleared to grow crops to feed confined animals in factory farms.[31] These crops are heavily contaminated with herbicides

---

27 John Robbins, *Diet for a New America: How Your Food Choices Affect Your Health, Your Happiness, and the Future of Life on Earth* (Walpole, NH: Stillpoint Publishing, 1987), 352.

28 John Vidal, "Protect Nature for World Economic Security, Warns UN Diodiversity Chief," *Guardian*, August 15, 2010, https://www.theguardian.com/environment/2010/aug/16/nature-economic-security.

29 Richard A. Oppenlander, *Food Choice and Sustainability: Why Buying Local, Eating Less Meat, and Taking Baby Steps Won't Work* (Minneapolis: Langdon Street, 2013).

30 Hiroko Tabuchi, Claire Rigny, and Jeremy White, "Amazon Deforestation, Once Tamed, Comes Roaring Back," *New York Times*, February 24, 2017, https://www.nytimes.com/2017/02/24/business/energy-environment/deforestation-brazil-bolivia-south-america.html?.

31 Will Tuttle, *The World Peace Diet: Eating for Spiritual Health and Social Harmony* (New York: Lantern, 2005), 185.

and pesticides, and in many cases these plants have been genetically engineered and contain GMOs that infiltrate our ecosystem.

7. Crops: The human world population in 1812 was 1 billion; 1.5 billion in 1912, and 7 billion in 2012; that number is projected to increase to 8 billion by 2021 and 9 billion by 2040.[32] We are growing enough plant- 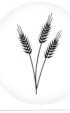 based food to feed 10 billion people,[33] but most of those people are not getting that food because it is being fed to livestock.[34] In the United States, 95 percent of the corn grown is fed to animals raised for food. Most of the soybeans grown in the world are not used to make tofu or soymilk for people, but are fed to livestock. Most of this feed has been genetically manipulated and is heavily laden with herbicides and pesticides.[35]

8. Fossil fuel depletion: It takes eleven times as much fossil fuel to produce a calorie of animal protein as it does to produce a calorie of grain protein.[36] Over one-third of all fossil fuels used in

32 Public Broadcasting System (PBS), "Human Numbers Through Time," PBS, https://www.pbs.org/wgbh/nova/worldbalance/numb-nf.html.

33 Eric Holt-Giménez, "We Already Grow Enough Food for 10 Billion People . . . and Still Can't End Hunger," Common Dreams, May 8, 2012, https://www.commondreams.org/views/2012/05/08/we-already-grow-enough-food-10-billion-people-and-still-cant-end-hunger.

34 FAO, Executive Summary, "Protein Sources for the Animal Feed Industry," FAO, 2003, http://www.fao.org/3/y5019e/y5019e00.htm.

35 United States Department of Agriculture Economic Research Service, https://www.ers.usda.gov.

36 International Panel on Climate Change (IPCC), United Nations, "AR5 Climate Change 2014: Impacts, Adaptation, and Vulnerability," IPCC, https://www.ipcc.ch/report/ar5/wg2.

the United States goes to raise animals for food.[37] The war in the Middle East, the war for oil, is being fought to fuel the meat and dairy industries in the United States. Agriculture accounts for more than twice as much of the U.S. energy budget as the military.[38]

Each day, a person who eats a vegan diet saves 1,100 gallons of water, 45 pounds of grain, 30 square feet of forested land, and at least one animal's life.[39]

A vegan diet is probably the single biggest way to reduce your impact on Planet Earth, not just greenhouse gases, but global acidification, eutrophication, land use, and water use. It is far bigger than cutting down on your flights or buying an electric car. [40]

—JOSEPH POORE, RESEARCHER, OXFORD UNIVERSITY

We are depriving ourselves and future generations of fresh water, clean air, and a toxin-free world. Our human technology is an extension of our unenlightened minds, which do not grasp the interconnectedness of life. As a result, we are rapidly contaminating all living things, present and future, by raising animals for food.

37 One Green Planet, "Facts on Animal Farming and the Environment," https://www .onegreenplanet.org/animalsandnature/facts-on-animal-farming-and-the-environment/.
38 Institute for Policy Studies, "Combat vs Climate: The Military and Climate Security Budgets Compared," https://ips-dc.org/wp-content/uploads/2016/09/CvsC-Report-1.pdf.
39 Lillie Ogden, "The Environmental Impact of a Meat-Based Diet," *Vegetarian Times*, April 4, 2007, https://www.vegetariantimes.com/life-garden/the-environmental-impact-of-a-meat-based-diet.
40 Damian Carrington, "Avoiding Meat and Dairy Is 'Single Biggest Way' to Reduce Your Impact on Earth," *Guardian*, May 31, 2018, http://www.theguardian.com/ environment/2018/may/31/avoiding-meat-and-dairy-is-single-biggest-way-to-reduce-your-impact-on-earth.

When left alone, undomesticated animals may not possess the technological skills and tools we have, but they may have something more vital that we do not: an innate intelligence and awareness of how to successfully coexist on Earth in the long term. Our environment is not becoming contaminated and barren because of wild animals. It is not because of them that we cannot drink from our rivers, lakes, and streams. Animals are naturally able to live with this planet and one another in ways that are sustainable and do not poison the air, soil, and water or destroy the habitats of other beings.

We, on the other hand, are destroying everyone else and ourselves with our destructive lack of awareness. Currently, the atrocities committed against animals in the name of human progress are the most important issues facing us all. With careful investigation, we will discover that most other issues plaguing us—from health crises to environmental woes to wars fought over land and oil—stem from it. Perhaps if we were to reverse our ways of relating to animals as mere things and instead began listening to them and observing how they live in harmony with the planet, we could learn some valuable lessons.

Yoga serves to awaken and remind us that we do know how to live in harmony with life. When we rediscover our own wildness, the shackles of our present culture will fall away, and we will find ourselves liberated from pretense and uncertainty. Yoga reveals to us the constraints and toxicity of our present culture. Yoga can show us the path to a renewed way of life and, ultimately, a way for us to stay alive.

In a larger context, *asana* refers to our relationship to the Earth, which includes the environment as well as all beings. But as is true of all "life" philosophies, both esoteric and exoteric components must be considered in order for us to develop deeper understanding of what it means to be alive. Yoga philosophy teaches that the reality we perceive as outside us is actually a reflection of what is inside us. This being so, the physical practice of asana allows us to deeply investigate, on a causal level, our relationship with the Earth and all other beings. It is through the investigation of our own body and mind that we discover within ourselves tendencies that we now see outside ourselves and want to change. Asana practice is indeed a very physical practice that respects the knowledge stored in the body and views the body not merely as something that carries the head around.

We cannot really "do" yoga, because Yoga is our natural state of being. Yoga refers to that enlightened state of living in harmony with all of existence. What we can do are certain practices that may reveal to us where we are resisting that natural state. Once these resistances are revealed or brought to the light of our conscious awareness, we have a better chance of letting them go. Asana practice like meditation is in essence a means of letting go of that which we are not to reveal who we truly are. This is why you can't "do" it. You can only let go and allow it. When resistances arise, we recognize and perceive them for what they truly are—or, we might say, where they are coming from.

Our bodies don't lie: They tell the story of our past. Our bodies are made up of the residue of all our past unresolved karmas. For something to be a yoga practice, it must help us purify these karmas. The practice of asana is a yoga practice because it allows us to resolve past relationships with others and clarify our perception of ourselves.

Therapeutically, asana has the power to heal emotional traumas and put the personality back into order so that we may function as happier, better-adjusted individuals. Essentially, however, the practice is designed to bring the individual beyond the healing of the body and mind and into a greater realization of the Self as whole, existing as a part of cosmic, eternal reality.

While we are engaged in certain asanas, particular physical and mental feelings arise. These feelings provide valuable insight into the nature of our personality—self. Ultimately, through the practice of asana, one can resolve the small self into the experience of the transcendent Self. This is possible because each time we engage in a particular asana, whether a standing asana like *trikonasana*, a forward bend like *paschimottanasana*, a twisting asana like *ardha matsyendrasana*, a backbend like *dhanurasana*, or an inversion like *sarvangasana*, we energetically relive past karmic experiences that have been stored in the cells and tissues of our physical body. (Refer to chapter 13, "Yoga on the Mat.")

Asana practice stimulates healing on many levels. Yes, it can help heal injuries and bring strength and flexibility to muscles and joints, but, spiritually, the practice of asana can release us from *avidya*, ignorance of who we really are. The practice of asana releases *pranic* (life-giving) energy, allowing it to flow through previously blocked subtle channels. When these channels flow with energy, we start to heal the disease of disconnection and begin to experience ourselves as much more than our physical body or personality self. We begin to experience ourselves as cosmic. What does that mean? It means we start to experience ourselves as part of a great whole, an interconnected eternal reality that transcends time and space. Wow! That's trippy!

Since yoga is a very practical science, before tripping out into the psychedelic mind-blowing reality of cosmic oneness, let us first look into the reality of relative experience: the day-to-day here and now. After all, there is truth to the ancient alchemical precept "As above, so below." To be free and make it to heaven, we must make heaven here on Earth. There is actually no other place to go but here. Everything we need to expand our consciousness is all right here and now. Asana is the key that can open up the doorway to the adventure waiting for us inside our own bodies, where our past, present, and future reside. By freeing our bodies of negative karmas (negative thoughts, words, and deeds), we awaken to the body as a potential vehicle for the Divine.

"The Divine" refers to that which is whole—that which is holy. When we are whole, we are able to become an instrument for peace, not destruction, because our actions arise out of the personal experience of the interconnectedness of all beings and things. Through our practice of asana, we build a holy (whole) body. As we free our bodies from fear, jealousy, and anger, we lift these negative emotions from the planetary atmosphere—which is, after all, only a reflection of what's going on inside us.

The actual physical substance of our bodies is derived from the food we eat. What or even whom we eat is decided by how we perceive and relate to others. When Patanjali tells us that if we want enlightenment, we should relate to others in a mutually beneficial way, he implies that we should not view others as objects for us to use—if, that is, we truly want enlightenment. When reflected on in this way, the sutra *sthira-sukham asanam* (PYS II.46) provides valuable insight into how to improve our relationships with the other animals with whom we share this planet. The asana practice we do on and off the mat provides us with profound opportunities to heal the planet and evolve our human consciousness.

If we are to survive as a species, we must make the transition from a culture based on slavery, exploitation, violence, and death to a way of life based on kindness, peace, harmony, and wholeness. The practice of yoga holds within it the means to dismantle our present culture and give us the know-how to build a new way of life. What could be a better place to start than with the question "What shall we eat today?"

Eating is the most fundamental basis for our life, as it creates and maintains our physical body, without which we would have no life. The choice to eat a vegan diet will do more to revolutionize our bodies, minds, and spirit and bring about world peace than any other single act, because it powerfully effects change in the outside world through enacting that change from deep within our own bodies. Such change will put into motion a profound planetary revolution, because it makes other-centeredness, not self-centeredness, the number-one priority. Up until this point in history, we have been members of a culture that gives priority to self-centeredness. For thousands of years, the enslaving and exploitation of animals has escalated and continued unquestioned, but now we are questioning. We are at the brink of a new level of consciousness that considers the well-being of the whole, not just a privileged few.

Asana refers to our connection to the Earth and other beings. When we allow ourselves to delve deeper into the meaning of *asana*, we realize the power this ancient practice has to heal the global crisis we are facing. Asana provides us a way to heal ourselves from the disease of disconnection through healing our relationships with others. When we feel physically, emotionally, mentally, and spiritually connected to nature and all other beings, the greater global healing can begin.

The Hopi Elders tell us that we have passed the eleventh hour (a time of reckoning) and that *now* is the hour. Therefore, we should deeply consider all our relationships, including what or whom we are eating and where and with whom we are living. The Hopi wisely tell us, "At this time in history, we are to take nothing personally, least of all ourselves, for the moment we do, our spiritual growth and journey come to a halt."

What could it mean to take oneself personally in such a way that causes one's spiritual growth to stop?

Our culture is essentially a domineering, herding culture. It is based on the enslavement of others, primarily other animal nations. It encourages us to seek self-gratification at the expense of others, even at the expense of the greater Earth community, mistakenly assuming that we can exist outside that community. The separation of spirit and body and of humanity and nature are results of the notion that the Earth belongs only to human beings. This ignorance (*avidya*) and egotism (*asmita*) lead to low self-esteem, and leave us feeling that what we do as individuals has little bearing on the whole. This feeling of insignificance represents the "personal" delusion that the Hopi Elders describe as the ultimate hindrance to our spiritual advancement.

Through communal yoga practice, as we experience the wonder of breathing together in a variety of ways, Self-confidence arises. Through chanting mantras and prayers, adding our voices to the choir, a greater sense of well-being develops. When we practice asana together, rhythmically moving in tune with breath and intention, we overcome debilitating estrangement, as we feel a part of a greater community. This unifying experience comes from a deep-rooted space of expansive yet inclusive consciousness, where all of existence is connected and pulsating with the joy of this wholeness, or holiness. The realization of unity is joyful and cannot be attained through hard struggle (working against something), but only through holy celebration.

Holy celebration is inclusive, as it embraces the whole community. Not one of us is an isolated case. Every action has tremendous impact on all of creation.

We must take responsibility for our behavior by looking into the possible outcome of our every exhaled breath, word spoken, and action taken, asking ourselves, "Is this contributing to the happiness and well-being of the greater community?" This, truly, is the key to unlocking our potential, making a boundless future on this Earth possible. If it is not, then have the courage to recognize that it is not a holy celebration, because it does not include the whole. Stop holding your breath and get yourself in tune. Breathe with one another, dismantling our present master/slave culture, and find a new way of living, based in the universal, unifying musical language of rhythm, harmony, and partnership.

The Hopi Elders inspire us to pulsate with the global community when they encourage us by saying, "The time of the lone wolf is over—gather yourselves! Banish the word *struggle* from your attitude and your vocabulary. All that you do now must be done in a sacred manner and in celebration. We are the ones we have been waiting for!"

CHAPTER 3

AHIMSA

Nonharming

Who will be the happiest person?
The one who brings happiness to others.
—SWAMI SATCHIDANANDA

Three things in human life are important.
The first is to be kind, the second is to be kind, and
the third is to be kind.
—HENRY JAMES

Ahimsa means "nonharming." What happens when you practice ahimsa long enough to become established in it?

ahiṁsā-pratiṣṭhāyāṁ tat-sannidhau vaira-tyāgaḥ
PYS II.35
When you stop harming others, others will cease to harm you.

ahimsa: nonharming, nonviolence
pratishthayam: being established or grounded in
tat: (in) that
sannidhau: presence
vaira: hostility
tyagah: give up, abandon

IN THE YOGA SUTRAS, PATANJALI GIVES US FIVE RECOM-
mendations, called *yamas*, for how we should treat
others if we want to attain Yoga—the realization of
the oneness of being. The first yama is *ahimsa*, which
means "nonharming."

Patanjali says that if you are seeing a multitude of
others and not One, then first and foremost, don't hurt
them! The yamas are directives for how we should
relate to others, not ourselves. Nonetheless, some contemporary yoga teachers interpet ahimsa as a directive
not to harm yourself. "Don't be aggressive in your
asana practice; be kind to your body," they say. Or else,
"Don't restrict your diet with extremes like veganism or
vegetarianism; it might harm you."

If Patanjali had been recommending ahimsa as a way
of treating oneself, he would have included it in his list of
niyamas, the observances one should maintain in regard
to oneself. The five niyamas are *saucha* (cleanliness),
santosha (contentment), *tapas* (discipline), *svadhyaya*
(study), and *ishvarapranidhana* (loving devotion to God).
None of these niyamas conflicts with ethical veganism,
while the yamas all support it. Not harming yourself is
a *result* of the practice of ahimsa, but if you limit your
practice of ahimsa to being kind to yourself, you will
deny yourself the ultimate benefit of yoga practice,
which is enlightenment. The fact that Patanjali placed
ahimsa as the first yama, and not among the niyamas,
or personal observances, seems vitally significant. So
much of the violence we see in the world today seems
to be out of our control, but what we choose to eat is
very much within our control.

We cannot change the suffering that has already happened in our lives, but future suffering can and should be avoided. A benefit of not causing others to suffer is that we will eventually, but inevitably, become free from suffering. We may mistakenly think that to refrain from harming another brings benefit only to that other, and not to ourselves. We often view extending kindness to animals as a form of charity. Many nonvegans may even look on vegans as depriving themselves of enjoyment by refraining from eating meat. But when you understand how karma works and how yoga works, you begin to realize that how you treat others *now* determines how much suffering or joy you experience in your future.

In the case of eating meat, fish, and dairy products, the suffering may occur relatively quickly in the form of health problems like heart disease, stroke, or cancer. But most often, the karmic seeds of violence, like all seeds, take time to gestate, sprout, and grow. One may not see the results of one's harmful actions right away. In fact, the negative seeds we plant now may not come to fruition until future lifetimes. There is no such thing as instant karma. If there were, eating a hamburger would cause a person to drop dead.

Through the practice of yoga and ethical veganism, we can realize that we were meant to live in harmony with all the other animals and all of life. We come to know that our physical bodies function better without having to instill fear into others and to kill them, and that there is no nutrient that we need that we can't get directly from plant sources or from sunlight. We will come to recognize that our old bodies can be transformed and become light and whole—holy bodies, used as vehicles to bring peace. We can truly become the peace we wish to see in the world, and all beings will rejoice in our presence and not fear and run away from us.

Nonharming is essential to the yogi because it creates the kind of karma that leads to eternal joy and happiness. According to the universal law of karma, if you cause harm to others, you will suffer the painful consequences of your actions. The yogi, realizing this, tries to cause the least amount of harm and suffering to others possible.

Compassion is an essential ingredient of ahimsa. Through compassion, you begin to see yourself in other beings. This helps you refrain from causing harm to them. Developing compassion does something more that is of special interest to the yogi. It trains the mind to see beyond outer differences of form. You begin to catch glimpses of the inner essence of other beings, which is happiness. You begin to see that every single creature desires happiness.

To develop compassion, examine the motives behind your actions. Are they selfish, or unselfish? Proclaiming that it is right to eat meat because it makes you healthier, for example, is *himsic*, or harmful, because it is an action stemming from a selfish motive. When you recognize that cows, pigs, and chickens, as well as all animals raised for food, want happiness just like you do, you recognize kindred souls. The distinction between you and other beings wears thin as awareness begins to dawn.

In truth, we all share consciousness, and harm inflicted on one being (be it animal or human) is felt by all, sooner or later. Some meat eaters like to advance the argument that vegetables have feelings, too, so what is the difference between eating chickens or carrots? The answer is simple: Patanjali gives ahimsa as a *practice*, meaning you do your best to cause the least amount of harm. The yogi strives to cause the least amount of harm possible, and it is clear that eating a vegan diet causes the least harm to the planet and all creatures.

Generally speaking, the disease of disconnection plagues the human condition. As a species, we are not at ease with ourselves—with our bodies, with our minds, or our feelings—nor are we at ease with others, whether human beings or other animals. We can be nervous, competitive, fearful, or worried. We crave respect and approval while simultaneously seeking dominance and power. We certainly aren't at ease with our environment and are constantly altering it to suit our needs or, more often, our desires, with little regard for how our actions impact others or the Earth. This "dis-ease" causes all sorts of problems. We are destroying ourselves, other animal species, and the planet in a misguided quest to find happiness or ease of being.

By enslaving other animals and abusing them through lifelong torture and degradation, we deprive them of freedom and happiness. How can we ourselves hope to be free or happy when our own lives are rooted in depriving others of the very thing we say we value most in life—the freedom to pursue happiness? If you want to bring more peace and happiness into your own life, the method is to stop causing violence and unhappiness in the lives of others.

We tell our children that "Might is not right," yet we throw that idea out the window when it comes to the everyday reality of using might to torture, humiliate, and kill the enslaved and confined animals we raise for food.

---

maitryādiṣu balāni PYS III.24
Through kindness, strength comes.

---

maitri: friendliness
adishu: et cetera (compassion, kindness)
balani: strength, power

This is a radical concept because it challenges our enculturation, which tells us that strength comes from weakening another. The fork can be a powerful weapon of mass destruction or a tool to lead a movement of peaceful coexistence. Eating a compassionate vegan diet will stop war and create peace in one's body, peace with the animal nations, and peace on Earth.

Indeed, it is very radical to be a vegan during these times! As Ingrid Newkirk reminds us, "Never be afraid of seeming radical. All the best people in history have always been radical." The word *radical*, like the word *radish*, derives from the root word *rad*, meaning "root." A radical is someone who attempts to dig to the root of a situation. Yogis have always been radical and were even considered heretical because Yoga philosophy says a mediator or priest is not necessary—*you* are a direct line to God. Yogis search for the root causes because they understand that effective change can occur only if you change a course of action from the causal point. Failure to understand this is why so many "liberating" revolutions of the past never elicited long-lasting positive change; they dealt only with surface symptoms, not the root causes of social and cultural problems.

If we are to discover lasting solutions for our contemporary problems, we should look at the circumstances that might have led to those problems. History shows us that the enslavement of animals served as the model for human slavery. First, animals were enslaved and exploited, and then it was not a far leap to begin treating humans "like animals" by enslaving and exploiting them as well.

In ancient India, the cow was economically essential. The word for *cow* became synonymous with many other terms used to describe the values of a culture founded on the exploitation of animals, primarily cattle. The goddess of nature, for instance, was called "the perfect cow" because she provided abundance for her worshipers. So, people came to look on nature as existing to be used and exploited. Cow herders from ancient times to the present have viewed the cow's existence as a means to provide human beings the four Ms: milk, meat, manure, and money.

In our quest for peace, it is valuable to recognize that the ancient wars in our culture's history were fought over disputes about animal ownership and the land needed to confine, graze, and grow crops to feed those animals. Interestingly, the Sanskrit word for *war* is *gavya*, literally meaning "the desire to fight for more cattle," and *gavishti* means "to be desirous of a fight." Both words come from the root *gav* or *go*, which means "cow." The domestication (enslaving) of cows led to war.

Yogis seek real and lasting liberation from suffering. The Sanskrit term *jivanmukti* reveals the philosophical idea that such liberation is possible even for a person who still has a physical body, rather than only after the body is shed. *Jiva* means "individual soul," and *mukti* means "liberation." Together, the words describe a liberated soul, a person who perceives himself or herself not as a separate individual, but as holy: one who is part of the whole of creation.

The *jivanmukta* experiences liberation—absolute freedom from all states of confinement and suffering—and wishes this for all beings. In Tibetan Buddhism, we find a similar idea in the concept of the *bodhisattva*: one who lives for the benefit of others and finds the highest joy in the happiness and liberation of others. *Yoga* means liberation. Slavery is contrary to liberation. We ourselves can never be free while taking away freedom from others. Through the practice of yoga, we begin to recognize ourselves as inseparable from the whole and realize that whatever we do to others, we ultimately do to ourselves.

Pratishthayam means "to become well established or grounded in a certain practice." If we want to live in a less violent world, we will have to give up violence ourselves. As we become less violent, the world around us becomes less violent. We cannot demand something that we ourselves are not willing to embody.

I once spoke to a well-known yoga teacher, who is not a vegan and who had told his students that veganism isn't an important aspect of the practice of yoga, about the subject of *ahimsa-pratishthayam* (being established in ahimsa). In a public statement at a yoga conference, he had said that it was not necessary to be a vegan in order to be established in ahimsa. I asked him whether he felt that a person could kill and eat an animal without causing the animal harm, which would be the only logical support for his statement. Instead of answering my question directly, he asked me whether I thought that Jesus and the Buddha were enlightened beings, and went on to tell me that neither of them were vegans. "How do you know that they were not vegans?" I asked. The reality is that no one knows for sure what they ate or didn't eat, but we certainly do know what *we* have been eating. We also know for sure whether we are living a peaceful, easeful life or one filled with violence and hostility.

Yoga is said to be the perfection of action by the removal of selfish motivation. Yogis use the world they live in and the way in which they interact with the world as a vehicle for transformation. A vegan diet is an informed, intelligent, and conscious way to act peacefully and selflessly each time we make a choice, because it takes into consideration the well-being of others as well as of ourselves.

The practice of yoga builds inner confidence. As we become more Self-confident, we become less fearful. We become less self-absorbed, and our ability to feel life all around allows us to hear what life is trying to communicate to us through nature. Speaking to us through the animals, trees, water, and air, the message is simple yet profound: All of life is interconnected. What we do to others affects us all.

When we begin to feel this, we can free ourselves from the false idea that the Earth belongs to us and instead use our lives to benefit others. In turn, we will become happy as we discover that the best way to uplift our own lives is to do all we can to uplift the lives of others. When we become well established in ahimsa, we live in such a way that all hostility ceases in our presence. Others will not harm us. They won't feel any animosity toward us or even think harmful thoughts about us. They will have no need to fear us. Animals will not cower or shake in our presence or fearfully run away from us. As we rid ourselves of violent tendencies, we purify the atmosphere surrounding us, which is but a projection of our inner ground of being.

CHAPTER 4

SATYA

Telling the Truth

If people knew the truth about how badly animals are treated in today's factory farms, if people knew how completely confined and immobilized these creatures are for their entire lives, if people knew how severe and unrelenting is the cruelty these animals are forced to endure, there would be change. If people knew, but too many of us choose to look the other way, to keep the veil in place, to remain unconscious and caught in the cultural trance. That way, we are more comfortable. That way is convenient. That way, we don't have to risk too much. This is how we keep ourselves asleep.

—JOHN ROBBINS

Satya means "truthfulness." What happens when one becomes established in truth?

satya-pratiṣṭhāyāṁ kriyā-phalāśrayatvam PYS II.36
When one does not defile one's speech with lies, the words one says are listened to and acted upon in a positive and immediate manner. The speaker will be able to say what they mean. What one says comes true.

satya: truth
pratishthayam: being established or grounded in
kriya: purifying action
phala: fruit, fruition, to come to pass
ashrayatvam: dependency

TREACHERY AND DECEIT WERE THE METHODS USED INITIALLY, thousands of years ago, to "domesticate" animals: Kill the parents, steal the baby, raise the orphan as if it were your own child. Thus, the baby bonds to you and grows up thinking it is part of your family. In this way, animals become dependent on you and trust you. You can easily exploit them—shear them, milk them, use them to make more babies. Then, when you have exhausted their usefulness to you, you kill them and—the final humiliation—eat them. This master/slave relationship began by deceiving baby animals and continues to this day.

When the natural bond that occurs between child and parent is dissolved, the child is not able to develop in a healthy way, and physical and psychological breakdowns are inevitable. The child remains dysfunctional, with a distorted perception of itself and others. This vulnerability makes it more easily manipulated by its oppressors. It is easier to manipulate others when you take away their personhood and see them as objects.

Life on a farm has never been a happy, healthy family experience for the animals. Even before the onset of factory farms, a farm was a place to raise and harvest animals. In agriculture, seeds are planted with the intention of reaping crops. Farm animals are treated like vegetables—as if they had the feelings of vegetables. Farms are breeding facilities, where rape and manipulation are common daily procedures. Farm animals are not allowed to develop normal relationships with others of their kind. The cow, pig, or ewe, for instance, will never actually have the chance to have a relationship with the male whose seed will father her children. She never even gets to have a relationship with the children she will give birth to. In most cases, she isn't even allowed to see or to touch her babies. She is kept chained to a stall looking straight ahead or, in the case of pigs, strapped down on her side on a concrete floor, immobilized as she gives birth and for the short time that she nurses her piglets.

The consumer is not told the truth about where food comes from. Instead, we are told lies. The meat and dairy industries spend millions of dollars on advertising to deceive us. Because these industries form the foundation of our economic system, government agencies also don't want the public to know. There are laws now protecting the animal-user industries from citizen scrutiny, and it is becoming harder and harder for animal rights groups to gain access to factory farms or slaughterhouses to film or take photographs. The few pictures and pieces of film footage that do exist and are available for public view are very threatening to the animal-user industries. Why? Because in our culture, seeing is believing, and these films and pictures show the truth, a truth that once seen is impossible to deny. We have a worldwide culture of denial when it comes to our treatment of animals. No one wants to talk about it. In fact, it is considered taboo to speak of it, as it may spoil one's appetite.

When advertising is employed to sell meat, milk, and eggs, pictures of happy animals enjoying family life on the farm are used: calves grazing beside their mothers in lush green fields or cute, fluffy baby chicks surrounding a doting mother hen in a country barnyard. The truth is that in factory farms, and in farms in general, mothers are never allowed to be with their babies. Images like this are false advertising. Although in our hearts we know the truth about how food animals are being used, we lie to ourselves. We perpetuate this untruth when we lie to our children and fail to encourage them to investigate the truth.

The more we lie to others, the more others will lie to us. Eventually, it becomes quite normal to communicate through lying, never really saying what we mean or doing what we say.

Advertising and various media use lies to keep us convinced that we must continue to enslave animals, to use and exploit them, and to eat their meat. This is a form of lying, a violation of the power of speech that destroys any chance of creating an atmosphere of satya, or truthfulness. This fragmentation of body, mind, and speech prevents the development of *dharana*, the ability of the mind to concentrate, and ultimately blocks the ability to meditate and merge with blissful transcendental reality. The ability to concentrate is a difficult enough practice for most people, regardless of whether they are vegans. Meat eaters who try to meditate have to deal with that obstacle, not to mention the paranoia and fear they experience as a result of terrorizing others.

Some meat eaters say they are peaceful people and would never hurt anyone—they didn't kill the animal; they're just eating what is convenient. This type of thinking is an example of how disempowered and disconnected most of the carnivorous members of our culture feel. They have been convinced that what they do doesn't really matter in the larger scheme of things. After all, it is only my lunch—just a piece of ham between two slices of bread; what harm could that do?

The fact is that when we buy the meat of an animal, we are the ones who have signed his or her death sentence. When a hit man is paid to murder someone, should we view the person who hired him as innocent and put the blame solely on the hired gun? If we are buying and eating meat and dairy products, then the slaughterhouse workers, meat packers, and factory farm workers are all working for us. If everyone in the world woke up tomorrow and refused to buy meat and dairy products, they would no longer be lucrative industries, which is the only reason that they exist.

Part of the process of transitioning into living more honestly is to hold yourself accountable for the things you do. When we stop blaming others for our actions, we take a giant step toward freeing ourselves from low self-esteem, which arises through continuously relinquishing our decision-making power to others.

I am very close with a family I have known for years. I have seen the children grow up. The parents have always respected my veganism, and when I arrive for a visit, the whole family adopts a vegan diet for at least the time I am with them. Normally, they aren't vegans and eat meat. One summer when I was visiting, one of the children, who was then a teenager, asked me why I am a vegan. I replied that I wanted to contribute to peace on this planet and not more violence. "So do I," he exclaimed. "You know me; I'm a very peaceful person, but I do eat meat. What does eating meat have to do with peace?"

"Eating animals is a violent act," I replied.

"Only if you kill the animal," he argued, "and I don't kill animals. I would never kill an animal or go hunting or hurt anyone. I just eat them, and someone else kills them."

"But you are the one paying for someone else to kill them. Doesn't that make you responsible?" I asked him.

"No," he replied, "because I don't buy the groceries. My parents do, not me."

This is not an isolated incident. Such feelings are commonplace in our hierarchical, structured societies. Accountability for one's actions is less important than doing what we are told or obediently going along with the crowd and never questioning. We are told over and over again that the actions of individuals are not important to the whole scheme.

The Perils of Obedience

PSYCHOLOGIST STANLEY MILGRAM CONDUCTED A FAMOUS experiment in obedience at Yale University in the

1960s. It was a study of how obedience, as a deeply ingrained behavior in our culture, can override ethics. The experiment measured the willingness of study participants to obey an authority figure, who instructed them to perform acts that conflicted with their personal conscience.

In his experiment, two people come to a psychology laboratory to take part in a study. One of them is designated a "teacher," the other a "learner." The experimenter explains that the study is concerned with the effects of punishment on learning. The learner is conducted into a room and strapped into a chair with what appears to be an electrode attached to his wrist. He is told that he will be read lists of simple word pairs by the teacher and that he will then be tested on his ability to remember the second word of a pair when he hears the first one again. Whenever he makes an error, the teacher will administer electric shocks of increasing intensity by pulling on a lever.

The teacher is a genuinely naive subject. The learner is actually an actor who receives no shock at all but pretends to. The learner sitting in the chair is in full view of the teacher. When the learner begins to miss words, the teacher pulls the lever to administer a shock.

When the actor/learner convulsed and appeared to be really suffering, and even screaming, the teacher would inevitably turn to the experimenter and ask to stop the experiment. The experimenter would always respond by insisting that the teacher continue with the experiment. The actor/learner would express pain more dramatically, and the teacher would again turn to the experimenter to ask whether the experiment should be halted. The experimenter would insist firmly that the teacher must complete the experiment.

Most of the subjects who participated in the experiment continued to shock the learner even while protesting to the experimenter that they felt what they were doing was unethical. They obeyed the experimenter in spite of their own feelings.

The experiments began in July 1961, three months after the start of the trial of Nazi war criminal Adolf Eichmann. Milgram said that he devised his experiment to question whether it was possible that Eichmann and his accomplices were just following orders.

"The question arises as to whether there is any connection between what we have studied in the laboratory and the forms of obedience we so deplored in the Nazi epoch," he wrote in the preface to his book, *Obedience to Authority*. "The essence of obedience consists in the fact that a person comes to view himself as the instrument for carrying out another person's wishes, and he therefore no longer regards himself as responsible for his actions."[41]

"Ordinary people, simply doing their jobs, and without any particular hostility on their part, can become agents in a terrible destructive process," Milgram wrote in a magazine article. "Moreover, even when the destructive effects of their work become patently clear, and they are asked to carry out actions

---

41 Stanley Milgram, *Obedience to Authority* (New York: HarperCollins, 1974), xviii.

incompatible with fundamental standards of morality, relatively few people have the resources needed to resist authority."[42]

"Even Eichmann was sickened when he toured the concentration camps, but he had only to sit at a desk and shuffle papers," he observed in *Obedience to Authority*. "At the same time, the man in the camp who actually dropped the Zyklon B into the gas chambers was able to justify his behavior on the ground that he was only following orders from above. Thus there is a fragmentation of the total human act. No one man decides to carry out the evil act and is confronted with its consequences. The person who assumes full responsibility for the act has evaporated. Perhaps this is the most common characteristic of socially organized evil in modern society."[43] In Milgram's experiment, 65 percent of the people tested did administer the highest voltage of electric shocks.

Interestingly, in a similar experiment conducted during the early sixties with rhesus monkeys (also known as macaques) instead of human subjects, the majority of the monkeys refrained from operating a device for securing food if it caused another monkey to suffer an electric shock.[44] One description of the experiment reads, "In a laboratory setting, macaques were fed if they were willing to pull a chain and

42 Stanley Milgram, "The Perils of Obedience," *Harper's*, December 1973, https://harpers.org/archive/1973/12/the-perils-of-obedience.

43 Stanley Milgram. *Obedience to Authority*, reprint ed. (New York: Harper Perennial, 2009), ii.

44 Jules Masserman, Stanley Wechkin, and William Terris, "Altruistic Behavior in Rhesus Monkeys," *American Journal of Psychiatry* 121(6) (1964): 584–585, https://ajp.psychiatryonline.org/doi/abs/10.1176/ajp.121.6.584.

electrically shock an unrelated macaque whose agony was in plain view through a one-way mirror. Otherwise, they starved. After learning the ropes, the monkeys frequently refused to pull the chain; in one experiment, only 13 percent would do so—87 percent preferred to go hungry. One macaque went without food for nearly two weeks rather than hurt its fellow. Macaques who had themselves been shocked in previous experiments were even less willing to pull the chain. The relative social status or gender of the macaques had little bearing on their reluctance to hurt others. . . . By conventional human standards, these macaques—who have never gone to Sunday school, never heard of the Ten Commandments, never squirmed through a single junior high school civics lesson—seem exemplary in their moral grounding and their courageous resistance to evil."45

In their behavior toward animals, all men are Nazis; for the animals, it is an eternal Treblinka.
—ISAAC BASHEVIS SINGER

Through the practices of yoga, we begin to connect to a place of conscience, which provides us with information about the possible outcome of our actions. To act from conscience is to act from independence—from being dependent inward. That place, which some call the heart, is our connection to the greater world, or the greater heart. When we act out of conscience, our

---

45 Carl Sagan and Ann Druyan. *Shadows of Forgotten Ancestors* (New York: Ballantine, 1992), 117.

actions are never merely self-serving; they serve the whole. As the Milgram experiment shows, our cultural conditioning can be so strong that it disconnects us from our heart, leading to a feeling of disempowerment. We can become programmed to act in a way that is fragmented and not true to ourselves. To do something because everybody else does it is not a good enough reason. To do it because we believe God told us to do it is not a good enough reason either. To live by violence and then to deny that you do is to live a lie. Living a lie causes a deep fissure in the human psyche. Yoga seeks to heal that fissure.

One of the ways you can tell if you are making progress in yoga, especially hatha yoga, is by observing your own voice. Through regular practice, you will find you are able to adjust the volume and pitch of your voice so you can be heard and understood, but most importantly, you will be able to say what you mean and mean what you say. When this happens, it is an indication that the disease of disconnection is beginning to be healed. You will be increasingly able to articulate with integrity from a place of deep universal connectedness rather than isolation.

It is thought of as quite normal these days for people to say one thing while thinking something else, and then do a contradictory third thing. One underlying cause of this symptom is that we have conditioned ourselves to disconnect from the reality of how we view and treat animals.

Most of us say we want peace, equality, and freedom for all, but our actions say something entirely different as we bite into a hamburger or order an ice cream cone, wear a fur coat to an antiwar demonstration, or serve hot dogs to our children. Once you become more aware, there's simply no way to not notice these everyday hypocrisies, these gaps in awareness justified by group behavior and the culture of "dis-ease."

By contemplating these issues with sincerity, you will realize that they are just an outgrowth of our ancient animal slave-based culture, which surrounds all of us at every turn. This disconnection between one's feelings or heartfelt beliefs and what one says and does stems from a patriarchal herding culture as old as Babylon. It may be interesting to note that Sumer, considered the cradle of Western civilization, is where both the herding of animals and the development of written language originated. The Sumerian cuneiform tablets are among the oldest written literature existing. This vast literature, mostly in poetic form, tells of man's conquest of animals and of nature and his move toward urban societies built on a hierarchical system of government, religion, and economics stemming from animal slavery.

For thousands of years, we have conditioned ourselves to do things we know in our hearts are morally wrong; yet we do them because we have been told to do so by the authority figures in our lives. We have been told that life is hard, and that in some situations we simply must buck up and do them anyway, even though they are unpleasant—like killing animals. We live a double standard: We don't want to tell our children where their food is coming from and don't want to do the killing, but we don't question the lie at the core of our abusive treatment of animals. The truth is that we don't have to hurt them, kill them, or eat them to be happy, healthy, and wise, but in order to become aware of that, we must decondition ourselves and explore ways to live and act from a place of the heart. As Stanley Milgram suggests, "It may be that we are puppets—controlled by the strings of society. But at least we are puppets with perception, with awareness. And perhaps our awareness is the first step to our liberation."

In *The Animals Film*, the filmmaker asked random people on the street the question "Do you like animals?" One woman gave the very revealing answer "Animals? I *love* animals!" Then he asked, "Do you eat animals?" The woman responded incredulously, "Eat animals? Yes. Doesn't everybody?" The filmmaker then asked, "But you said you loved animals. Is there a contradiction there?" To which the woman replied, "Well, I'd like to live by my principles, but I don't, 'cause we gotta eat, don't we?"

The industries that exploit animals create self-serving euphemisms to conceal the truth of their actions. A survey of your local supermarket will turn up such terms as "humanely slaughtered" and "raised according to animal welfare standards" on packages of meat and cartons of eggs. If you look up *humane* in a dictionary, you will find a definition like "characterized by compassion, sympathy, kindness, mercy, or consideration for other human beings or animals." If you look up *welfare*, you might find "concerned for another's health, happiness, and well-being."

These industries have become experts at what Tom Regan refers to as "Humpty-Dumpty talk" in his book *Empty Cages*.46 In Lewis Carroll's classic *Through the Looking Glass*, when Alice comes across the egg, Humpty-Dumpty, they have a conversation in which Alice becomes frustrated with Humpty's way of defining things. He uses words to mean something totally different from what they actually mean. When Alice confronts him with this, he says, "When I use a word, it means just what I choose it to mean—neither more nor less."

We, in turn, use Humpty-Dumpty talk to lie to our children about what we are really feeding them, and they grow up learning that no one has to be honest about anything. They are given the message that denial, not honesty, is valued and should be cultivated. We override our children's natural sense of compassion by showing them pictures on packages of meat of cute animals dressed up and happy, or cartoons of pigs eating ribs, cows offering ice cream sundaes, or smiling burgers bouncing up and down in a burger garden saying, "Eat me, please!"

If we don't want to be taken in by the lies people tell us, we can begin to examine our own speech and ask ourselves if we are really saying what we mean. If we say we want peace on Earth, are we willing to do what is necessary to create it? Are we willing to speak

---

46 Tom Regan. *Empty Cages: Facing the Challenge of Animal Rights* (Oxford: Rowman & Littlefield, 2004), 78.

truthfully at every turn and be honest with others and ourselves? This is difficult work, but once begun, it becomes easier with practice. It is, like yoga itself, a lifelong effort.

If we want others to speak well of us, are we willing to stop gossiping, judging, and blaming others? True or not, we humans tend to assume we are superior to other animals because we have the ability to speak. Yet scientists have observed that other animals can and do speak, but in languages that we cannot understand. All of nature communicates. Why is it that we cannot hear what she is saying? We want so much for others to hear us. Half the effort in speaking truthfully lies in listening well. Are we listening to the anguished cries of the animals in factory farms or the shrieks of the slaughtered?

If we grew up eating meat and dairy products, then our own bodies have been formed from animals whose voices we had a hand in silencing when they were locked away to cry on their own in lonely warehouses and had their throats cut at the time of slaughter. How might this have an impact on our own ability to speak truthfully— and to be heard?

I have observed in my years of teaching yoga that many students are quite shy when it comes to speaking in public, let alone singing or chanting mantras. Shyness could be seen as a form of vanity because it exists when we are thinking of ourselves and our feelings and not the feelings of the people in front of us. It lacks empathy and comes from a deep self-consciousness and self-absorption, which stems from feeling separate.

Why do so many of us feel so shy? Musician and activist Michael Franti says that the biggest fear people have is the fear of having to speak in public and that fear is second only to the fear of having to sing in public. But why? Some people blame early childhood experiences; perhaps teachers, parents, or siblings silenced them with harsh judgmental words like "Shut up! You can't carry a tune," or "You're no Pavarotti or Elvis Presley!" These types of experiences are by no means rare in our culture but might be viewed as symptoms rather than causes.

If we look more deeply at some of our more indigenous human relatives who have not distanced themselves so far from nature and live more closely with wild animals, we find societies in which singing and dancing are considered normal everyday activities for every member of the tribe. Within so-called uncivilized tribal societies, singing and dancing is not a performance art or "dis-play" but is engaged in as actual play—a form of communication with life, rather than as a commodity to be taken to the market place. Have we traded our natural musical abilities, which would allow us to express ourselves freely or even wildly in song and dance, for a more domesticated version of ourselves?

Most of us unconsciously accept that our "civilized" way of life is better than the wild, savage version. After all, we have been told this over and over again over countless lifetimes. We, in turn, pass on these unexamined assumptions to our children, unaware that we may be lying to them and to ourselves. We don't question the results of a 10,000-year war on animals, nature, and all that is wild. Yet our domesticated civilized life has been bought at great cost not only to nature and the animals but also to ourselves. As we have domesticated animals and robbed them of their wildness, we have become domesticated ourselves and lost our natural ability to be expressive and spontaneous. We have become nervous, neurotic, self-conscious, and—at the same time—vain and arrogant.

I once visited an animal sanctuary in South Carolina, which rescues exotic animals from abusive situations in circuses, sideshows, theme parks, and the like and provides them with a fairly safe haven. I say "fairly" because they are still captive, but at least they are spared the degradation of travel and performance. When I first arrived, the owner was very excited to give me a tour and introduce me to some of the lions, tigers, elephants, baboons, chimpanzees, zebras, bears, wolves, and mountain lions (to name but a few). He took me to the "nursery" to show me the babies and said, "My commitment is to, number one, help these animals get over their fear of humans and, number two, help them get over their fear of each other."

The nursery was a fenced-in yard with a large barn attached. Every morning, he brought all the babies together to play and returned them to their parents in the afternoon. I was immediately greeted by two five-month-old tigers, who ran to me, tumbling over themselves in the process. The tigers shared their play space with a baby mountain lion, a baby bear named Ursula, and Bambina, a gentle, big-eyed, two-month-old fawn. They all seemed to be quite chummy with one another, but that wasn't the most extraordinary thing that struck me as I sat on the ground surrounded by these furry children. It was the cacophony of voices: They all seemed to be speaking at once. From my perspective, it appeared that they were either in a continuous dialogue with one another, mumbling to themselves, or just talking and singing for the sake of it.

I was literally dumbstruck, as I had ignorantly assumed that all animals were basically mute and only let out a howl, bark, or meow on occasion, like the pet dogs and cats I had known (except for the Siamese cats I have had the privilege of living with, who normally do engage in lengthy conversation and commentary on life).

From this experience, I gained an insight about how our domestication of animals and its repression of all their natural tendencies might have led to a repression of their voices, causing them to become mute. The common practice used in all situations where there is slavery is to separate the babies from their parents while they are very young. The babies are not allowed to develop communication and speaking skills, as they would have if they had been allowed to be tutored by their parents. Wild animals, in contrast, talk a lot and without inhibition. Could there be a connection between how we have treated animals and our own inability to speak or sing freely?

In his book *Dominion*, Matthew Scully recounts, "I think of a fellow I know, in many respects devout and conscientious, who recently tried to shock me with a story about a laboratory (in Indiana, as I recall) where, to silence the yapping of some sixty dogs, the researchers cut out the vocal cords of each one. The dogs still try to bark, my colleague told me, as if relating some hilarious punchline, only it looks like someone has pressed the mute button, and now the scientists can go about their work in peace and quiet. Where does this spirit come from, that can laugh at such a thing?"[47]

As yoga practitioners, we come to a time in our lives when we begin to question whether what we have been told is true, including the assumptions we hold about ourselves and the world around us. The fact that you have begun a yoga practice is evidence that you have the courage to embark on a deep self-reflective quest. Through such self-reflection, you will encounter blockages to your creativity and self-expression. It is during those crucial moments, while engaged in asana or meditation practice, that it is important not to harbor negative thoughts. Do not blame others or feel guilty, inadequate, or overwhelmed. Instead, allow the past karmic residue to arise, and let it go with each passing breath. Through steady practice (abhyasa), you will experience for yourself what is true, and all the lies you have been told, even those you have told, will fade away in the light of the greater truth of your true potential.

As we embrace the practice of satya, our speech becomes purified, and we are able to fearlessly say what we mean and mean what we say. Others cease lying

47 Matthew Scully. *Dominion: The Power of Man, the Suffering of Animals, and the Call to Mercy* (New York: St. Martin's, 2002), 18.

to us and begin to perceive us as people with integrity; they listen to us and take our words seriously. What we say comes true. As Mahatma Gandhi suggested, we "become the change we wish to see in the world."

CHAPTER 5

ASTEYA

Nonstealing

Yoga is that state where you are missing nothing.
—SHRI BRAHMANANDA SARASVATI

Asteya means "not to steal." What happens when one becomes established in asteya?

asteya-pratiṣṭhāyāṁ sarva-ratnopasthānam PYS II.37
When one stops stealing from others, prosperity (material, mental, and spiritual) appears.

asteya: nonstealing
pratishthayam: being established or grounded in
sarva: all
ratna: jewels, money, wealth, prosperity
upasthanam: appear or approach

THE MEAT, DAIRY, AND FASHION INDUSTRIES ARE FOUNDED on stealing—stealing milk intended for a mother's new baby, stealing wool intended to keep someone warm, stealing skin and fur intended to be worn by the being who was born into that skin. To confine an animal for its entire life is to steal its life. To kill and eat animals is to steal their lives from them. The meat and dairy industries have successfully convinced us not to stop to think that animals may have their own purpose for living that doesn't include being exploited and used up by us, their human enslavers.

Through the practice of yoga, you come to feel confident and develop a feeling of wholeness and completeness; you are not likely to feel deprived or less than. People steal because they feel deprived. They try to make up for their deficits by depriving others. Our culture teaches us that if we have the money to pay for it, we can have it. We can own land or animals if we pay for them. We used to be able to own humans, if we paid for them, until we came to understand that human slavery is wrong. Now we are on the brink of realizing that enslaving animals is wrong.

Our present culture began roughly 10,000 years ago in Sumer, in the area currently known as Iraq. At that time, people began to domesticate animals. Dogs were the first, enslaved to help with hunting. Domestication is a polite way of describing enslavement. The first animals to be enslaved and exploited for food were sheep and goats. Before domestication, these animals were wild, living harmoniously with the rest of the natural world, as all wild animals know how to do. Once enslaved, the only purpose accorded to them by their captors was to be exploited by human beings, who controlled every aspect of their lives—deciding where they lived, whom they lived with, what they ate, and when they would die. These humans milked, sheared, bred, and ate the animals, considering them property. A person's wealth, power, and status came to be equated with the number of animals he owned and dominated.

After goats and sheep, cows were the next wild animals to be enslaved. It's funny, but most of us don't think of cows as once being wild animals. This shows something about how ingrained the notion of owning and eating animals has become. It seems normal to confine "barnyard animals," as if it has always been that way—as if they were born to live on farms as slaves. There is a growing movement of people today who feel that factory farms are wrong, but these people do not feel the same way about eating, milking, and exploiting animals in general. They would like to revert to the ideal of the small family-owned farm, not realizing that the small farm is, in essence, the factory farm on a smaller scale: a place where animals are fattened for slaughter. I feel that it is time for us to question the basic cultural assumption that animals exist as slaves to be exploited by us. If we ourselves want to get to the root cause of many of our problems today, we might start by critically examining the concept of the farm.

Our English word *capital* comes from the Latin word *capita*, which means "head," referring to heads of cattle, sheep, or goats. The first capitalists fought wars over land and livestock, and we are still fighting.

According to Will Tuttle's book *The World Peace Diet*, "Livestock in the ancient herding cultures thus defined the value of gold and silver—food animals were the fundamental standard of wealth and power. This fact gives us insight into the political might of the ranching and dairy industries that continues to this day."[48] In fact, our modern-day term "stock market" is derived from the ancient practice of trading livestock as commodities.

In the way that organisms depend on genes to keep their traits alive and embodied, a culture relies on *memes*. A meme is an idea, behavior, style, or trend that spreads from person to person within a culture. When an idea or behavior becomes integrated into the minds and habits of a people, it becomes perceived unquestionably as "normal" and as "always having been this way—everybody does it." The exploitation of animals has become a meme. When you understand this, you can take the first step in freeing yourself from the propaganda of your culture. The practices of yoga help us to question these long-standing habits.

An important meme for our present culture is "the Earth belongs to us," implying that it is the right of human beings to exploit the Earth and all other beings. Yoga holds the power to dismantle our present culture and gives us the means to learn how to live harmoniously with nature. The word *exploitation* means "treatment with little regard for the welfare, benefit, or happiness of the other." We live in a culture in which most everyone agrees that it is okay to enslave animals and that it is okay to eat them. In fact, it is expected of us that we eat them, and it is considered strange to question this expectation.

The first mention of memes is found in ancient Sumerian texts, which are some of the oldest surviving

---

48 Tuttle, *The World Peace Diet*, 19.

texts of our present culture. In Sumerian mythology, the moon goddess, Inanna, daughter of the sun, was said to have stolen the memes from her father and used them to build a civilization. The first city she built was called Uruk, and it existed about 150 miles from present-day Baghdad. Archaeologists have discovered cuneiform tablets and cylindrical stone seals in this area. These seals are carved with pictures, some of which depict warriors in battle, shepherds, and cattle. Sumeria was a "land of milk and honey," an ancient meat-eating and milk-drinking civilization founded on the enslavement of animals.

Our modern cities are based on the Sumerian meme, a way of life in which human beings' desires are given paramount importance and all other forms of life are perceived to exist primarily to be exploited by humans. But yoga has always existed in opposition to the rules, regulations, and cultural norms of the times in which it is practiced. The natural laws of beauty and harmony are the laws of the yogi. Yogis have always rejected the ways of civilization, with its degrading, imposing moral codes that, rather than respecting nature, are founded on taming and manipulating her. Yoga is based on the love of nature and the pursuit of ecstasy. The yogi understands that there is an innate order to wildness and that liberation comes through the blessings of the Divine Goddess, who is Mother Nature. Shiva, who is said to have been the first teacher of yoga, is a wild man who lives in the forest with the animals. He is called *Pashupati*, which means "protector of the animals." You could say that Shiva was the first environmental/animal rights activist.

The moral codes of urban society would have us fear wildness, telling us it is chaotic. In truth, nature is anything but chaotic—she operates in a very organized fashion.

Ritual animal sacrifice was a product of a culture that kept domesticated animals as slaves to be used for exploitation. In India, yogis sought refuge in the forest, where they could live close to nature and keep their distance from such barbaric rites, preferring to seek communion with the Divine through direct means. Yogis were considered heretics for rejecting the idea that it was necessary to pay an intermediary to recite spells over the burning bodies of slain animal victims in order to connect with divinity. In *Gods of Love and Ecstasy: The Traditions of Shiva and Dionysus*, author Alain Daniélou notes, "Throughout the course of history, urban and industrial societies—those exploiters and destroyers of the natural world—have been opposed to any ecological or mystical approach to the liberation of man and his happiness."[49]

Yoga is a tantric practice—worshiping the Goddess in the form of nature. Its methods align us with rather than oppose the forces of nature. Rejecting cultural pressure to despise the body and look on it as animalistic, needing to be clothed and tamed, yogis value the physical body as a potential vehicle for direct ecstatic transcendental communion with the Divine.

In our present time, we may not think we are stealing from others when we eat meat and dairy

49 Alain Daniélou, *Gods of Love and Ecstasy: The Traditions of Shiva and Dionysus* (Rochester, NY: Inner Traditions, 1992), 16.

products because we have been deluded into thinking that those others, the animal slaves, exist for our benefit and that if we pay at the supermarket or the restaurant, we are entitled to them. But the ultimate truth is that the animals never entered into any agreement to be bought and sold. We have been stealing their lives for our own selfish reasons. According to Patanjali, this is not conducive to our material, mental, and spiritual prosperity. This is how karma works. When we steal, we set into motion dire karmic consequences that affect our future well-being.

When someone says to me, "If people choose to eat meat, it is their business. We should not interfere, and we should be tolerant and accommodating of their dietary preferences," I have to say that whatever any of us does affects us all. When someone eats meat, it affects all of us because of the terrible environmental impact of the meat and dairy industries on the planet. By eating meat, we are not only stealing the lives and happiness of billions of animals, we are also stealing fresh water and clean air from future generations who will be born into this world.

At a yoga conference, I was having dinner with some colleagues when a certain dish was passed to me. Just before I was about to spoon out a portion onto my plate, someone remarked, "Oh, you probably won't want to eat that. It has butter and cheese in it." A yoga teacher sitting next to me asked, "What? You don't eat milk products? That's not very yogic, is it? What's wrong with milk? You can still be a vegetarian and drink milk, can't you? Isn't it more cruel to the cows not to milk them?"

I responded, "Milk is the fluid that comes from the breasts of a female cow when she is pregnant or has just given birth to a baby. The milk her body is producing is intended for her baby. I think it is in keeping with the principles of yoga to be kind (*ahimsa*) and not to steal from another (*asteya*) what is not intended for you."

"But," my friend continued, "drinking milk is better than eating flesh. At least no animal is being killed for you to drink milk."

"When her milk production drops," I replied, "every dairy cow ends up at the slaughterhouse."

"No, that's not true!" my friend emphatically stated.

"What do you think happens to a cow who can't produce milk anymore?" I asked.

"Well, I am sure the cow eventually dies, and then they probably bury her," she replied.

It would be nice to believe that dairy cows live to a ripe old age, die peacefully, and are buried by their caretakers, but the truth is, most dairy cows are destined, eventually, for the slaughterhouse.

Before you eat something, put it to the "**SOS**" test, devised by Ingrid Newkirk. Ask yourself this question: "Was anyone **S**laughtered **O**r **S**tolen from to provide this food for me?" If the answer is yes, don't eat it.

Can we afford to care about the suffering of animals when so many human beings are starving? Yes, not only because caring about animals does not preclude caring about human beings but also because veganism is of direct benefit to the planet and to reducing starvation around the world. A human child dies of malnutrition every two seconds on this planet, yet it takes 12–20 pounds of grain to produce 1 pound of meat. If just 10 percent of American meat eaters adopted a vegan diet, there would be 12 million more tons of grain to feed to humans—enough to support the sixty million people who starve to death each year.[50] When we come to understand the true benefits that come from the practice of asteya—nonstealing—the means to abolish human starvation will be realized, and all will have enough to eat.

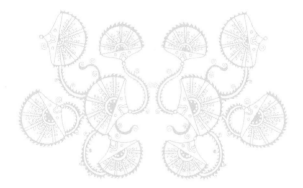

50 Rebecca Saltzberg, "The Steps to End World Hunger," *Down to Earth*, https://www. downtoearth.org/articles/2009-03/29/steps-to-end-world-hunger.

CHAPTER 6

BRAHMACHARYA

Good Sex

At the Animal Research Institute, we are trying to breed animals without legs and chickens without feathers.
—ROBB S. GOWE, DIRECTOR OF THE ANIMAL RESEARCH INSTITUTE, AGRICULTURE CANADA, SPEAKING AT AN AGRICULTURAL CONFERENCE IN OTTAWA[51]

Brahmacharya means "to respect the creative power of sex and not abuse it by manipulating others sexually." What happens when one becomes established in brahmacharya?

brahmacharya-pratiṣṭhāyāṁ vīrya-lābhaḥ PYS II.38
When one does not misuse sexual energy, one obtains enduring vitality, resulting in good health.

brahmacharya: not misusing sex
(**brahma:** the creative principle, God as creator +
charya: vehicle or means to)
pratishthayam: being established or grounded in
virya: vigor, vitality
labhah: gained

---

51 Jim Mason and Peter Singer. *Animal Factories* (New York: Harmony, 1990), 35.

BRAHMACHARYA IS A WAY TO GET TO GOD—A WAY TO arrive at the creative essence of the universe. It has sometimes been translated as "continence" or "chastity," which I feel has led to a lot of misunderstanding in regard to how to practice this yama. To practice *brahmacharya* is to understand the potential of sexual energy, which is the essence of all physical and psychological forces. Sex is the power that creates life. When sexual energy is directed wisely, it becomes a means to transcend separateness, or otherness. When sexual energy is used to exploit, manipulate, or humiliate another, however, it propels us into deeper separation and ignorance (*avidya*). Human beings routinely do this to the other species we confine in breeding facilities on farms. The sexual abuse of animals is ingrained in our culture, and it expresses itself in the practice of breeding, genetic manipulation, castration, artificial insemination, forced pregnancy, routine rape, and child abuse, which all fall under the category of animal husbandry.

Animals in factory as well as on most farms are not allowed to develop normal sexual relationships with others of their own species. Most confined animals never even see a member of the opposite sex of their own kind. All the animals born in factory farms have come from mothers who have been artificially inseminated. These mothers will be repeatedly raped by human farmhands and forced to become pregnant over and over again until their fertility wanes, at which point they will be slaughtered and eaten. Male animals chosen to be sperm donors are used and abused, live in constant frustration, and in the end, are slaughtered as well.

A male hog who is used as a sperm donor, for instance, is tethered and held in place while farm workers excite him by rubbing and massaging his testicles, penis, and foreskin until he is ready to ejaculate. The farm worker must then grab the animal's penis and aim it into a plastic "collection" tube.

Such practices are violent, crass, and degrading to animals, and dehumanizing for the farm workers paid to do this work. The way these animals are routinely sexually abused reveals just how disconnected we have become from the natural world and the beauty and miracle of life. Some may feel that using the word *rape* to describe what happens to animals might be anthropomorphizing. But by looking more closely at the word, we may come to recognize its broader implications. The Latin root of the word is *rapere*, meaning "take by force, aggressively violate sexually, disgrace, or ravage." Therefore, *rape* is the appropriate term to use for the abuse being perpetrated on defenseless enslaved animals confined to farms.

Like us, animals are people, too, endowed with souls, personalities, and the ability to feel pain, physical as well as emotional. We might do well to keep in mind that human beings are actually animals, too—we are one species among many. When we free ourselves from our prejudice against other animals, we will begin to see them as living beings deserving of rights just as we are. Therefore, just as we would not condone exploiting pregnant and lactating women for their milk, we should not condone this treatment of animals. If we look at it from this perceptive, eating meat, eggs, and dairy products could be seen as a feminist issue, for if we believe in women's rights, we cannot condone and support the way female animals are exploited for what their bodies can produce. Most of the animals in our factory farms are female because they are the most exploitable, as they can provide eggs or milk as well as more babies.

This has historically been the case in agriculture. Our culture is based on the exploitation of the feminine (Mother Nature), and so the eating of meat, eggs, and dairy products is an integral part of our system. If we feel that women should be treated fairly, we must extend our desire for women's liberation to all females regardless of race, religion, or *species*. Yoga teaches us that what we do to others, we ultimately do to ourselves. If we do not respect the rights of females of other species, how can we expect to successfully liberate human females?

Let's examine what happens to an average dairy cow on today's farms.

She lives in a tiny stall with a concrete floor in an indoor "milk facility" and has never seen the sun or stepped on ground or grass. She is not even a year old, yet she has just given birth to her first calf a few hours ago, which wasn't easy while being chained by the neck. She had tried to lie down, but it was hard, and harder to get back up. Now, the tethering chain makes it difficult for her to get close to her baby—but the baby is there, she knows. The baby is nursing, but not for long. Within hours, men come to take her baby. They shout at her, using harsh words. She tries to turn her head to see what is happening, but the chain prevents her from moving. She cries out to her baby, who cries back. In a few minutes, she no longer hears the cries of her newborn. He is in a truck being driven to a "veal facility," and his cries are out of her range of hearing. She is left in her place, her milk dripping from her breasts.

The milking machine now mechanically moves into place and clamps onto her nipples, sucking her and emptying her of the vital life force, which was intended for her baby. The machine will come again two more times today and most every day after that. She is crying and desperate to know what has happened to her baby. She becomes sad and depressed for weeks.

Soon after, a farm worker returns to her stall. She is chained, unable to turn around, defenseless when he inseminates her. She has given birth, had her baby stolen from her, been milked excessively by a machine, and now she is being raped again. The worker first inserts his hand, then forces his arm up to his elbow, into her vagina to open it up and locate her uterus. He then lodges the inseminator, a long, stainless-steel syringe, inside her and pumps sperm into her to impregnate her. She is now lactating and pregnant. She has to be pregnant or lactating to be able to produce milk, and in our culture, producing milk is the reason for her existence. She is viewed as a milk machine, a slave, one of billions of cows confined in factory-farm concentration camps.

In 1940, the average milk cow in the United States produced 2 tons of milk per year. Today a dairy cow, thanks to artificial insemination, genetic engineering, antibiotics, growth hormones, and cheap "enriched" feed, produces up to 10 tons per year. To get a cow to produce that much milk is unnatural and requires drastic measures. A cow by nature is vegan, eating only plant foods, so to be able to produce the amount of milk that will turn a profit, she is force-fed the flesh of other animals. It is common practice on today's farms to feed chickens, turkeys, cows, pigs, sheep, and goats "enriched" feed made of genetically modified corn, soy, oats, or wheat and laced with the rendered remains of slaughtered animals. Rendered meat by-products contain not only the body parts of animals raised in factory farms (chickens, turkeys, pigs, sheep, goats, and cows) but also dead animals collected from laboratories, zoos, schools, city shelters, circuses, and puppy and kitten mills; road kill; and fish. Most of the fish caught by commercial trawlers is not eaten by humans but fed to livestock. The U.S. Food and Drug Administration assures us that since the outbreaks of bovine spongiform encephalopathy (BSE, or mad cow disease), the "enriched" feed fed to cows doesn't include other cows in the recipe; nevertheless, it still includes their brains and spinal cords.[52]

Once pregnant again, the dairy cow remains chained by the neck in her stall with nothing to do but stand on concrete day in and day out, enduring the milking machine that empties her several times a day,

---

52 Dave Syverson, "Questions and Answers Concerning Pet Food Regulations," Association of American Feed Control Officials, Aug. 18 2008, https://petfood.aafco.org/Portals/1/pdf/q_and_a_petfood_regs.pdf.

until the last two months of her pregnancy, when she won't be milked. Even though she just stands there, her body is working very hard to produce all that milk and carry a baby in her womb. The amount of energy she expends is equivalent to what a human would use if he were to jog for six hours every day.[53] But this cow isn't able to get any exercise, as she can't move, and her udders become so full that they drag on the concrete floor and are heavy, swollen, and painful. The milking machine cuts her sometimes and causes sores; at other times, it gives her an electric shock, which makes her continuously afraid and anxious.

She is impregnated every year until she is four years old. By that time, she is physically and emotionally broken and her milk production is waning, so she is scheduled to be taken off the milking machine.

Farm workers arrive, and for the first time in her life, they unchain her from her stall. They push her roughly, trying to get her out of her stall. She is afraid and confused, and her legs are sore. The men are forcing her to walk. She has never walked before and doesn't know what is expected of her. The workers push and shove her and prod her with a device that gives her an electric shock. Somehow, she manages to get out of the building. This is also happening to many of the other cows who have been in the building with her for the last four years. They are all loaded into a large truck. It is very crowded in the truck, and all of them are

---

53 C. David Coats. *Old MacDonald's Factory Farm: The Myth of the Traditional Farm and the Shocking Truth About Animal Suffering in Today's Agribusiness* (New York: Continuum, 1989) 55.

afraid. They peer through the slats in the sides of the truck. They have never seen the light of day; they have never seen anything except the inside of their stall in the milking facility. It is cold, and their udders are full of milk and very sore. They travel for a long time, as it becomes dark and then light again. The truck stops, and when the door opens, the men pull and push them out of the truck. The cows hear screaming and smell blood; they become terrified. The more scared they become, the more violent and impatient the men are, yanking and kicking them to move them faster. Some of the cows collapse, their legs just giving out on them. The men kick and use electric prods to shock these downed cows into standing up and walking. If that doesn't work, they may use a hose to force water up their noses to try to get them to stand and walk into the slaughterhouse.

The cow somehow makes it into the new building, but she senses that it is a place of death. She can't escape, and as before, she is unable to turn around. As a worker tries to shoot a steel pellet into her head, she moves, and instead, he shoots her in her left eye. She is shackled and yanked up into the air, her heavy body hanging from one leg. She is seeing so much suffering and death. She is crying, but no one seems to be listening. A man with a large sharp—or worse, dull—knife cuts her throat, shoves his hand into this cruel wound, and pulls out her trachea. She struggles to get free. She is conscious and aware, but there is no one to help her. She hangs upside down, bleeding to death. Next, some other men begin to cut and dismember her body. As they cut into her abdomen, the baby she has been carrying in her womb falls out onto the killing floor.

Her body, once viewed as a milking machine, is now just so much meat and will most likely end up as cheap hamburger in a fast-food restaurant. The baby she was carrying? Its body will be skinned, and the soft leather will be sold as expensive calfskin.

As many former workers have verified, the animal-user industries consider abuse normal in factory farms and slaughterhouses. There are many incidences of slaughterhouse workers being caught on undercover film sexually abusing the animals whom they are also killing and dismembering. There are also incidences of farm workers sexually abusing confined and tethered animals in factory farms. As most animals are tethered (held in place by ropes, chains, or straps), they are acutely vulnerable to abuse. Many female pigs are strapped down to a concrete floor, unable to move. Veal calves, having been taken away from their mothers at birth and confined in small crates, are desperate to suck and will suck on anything. Some farm workers take advantage of these helpless baby animals. These are not a few isolated incidences—it is widespread.[54] The only difference between sexually abusing an animal in a slaughterhouse and raping an animal confined in a factory farm is that what happens to the animal in the factory farm is commonly accepted and excused as part of the necessary business of breeding, and what goes on in the slaughterhouses is considered "not procedure."

---

54 To see acts like these caught on film, visit https://www.peta.org or https://www.hsus.org.

Either way, the same thing is going on—an animal is being brutally and intimately violated without his or her consent.

Is there any reason to doubt the connection between widespread pornography and this kind of unspeakable animal exploitation? Both are rooted in the blind ambition to dominate—the antithesis of a yogi's instinct and pursuit. Both are considered acceptable, tolerated, and possibly even "normal" within our culture, one that is based on the degradation of the feminine and disconnection from the sacredness of life.

Consider the snuff film—the epitome of perverse pornography. The finale is the murder of a woman, preferably pregnant, her abdomen sliced open and her uterus cut out. Pornography is just a symptom of a culture in which the subjugation, rape, and dismembering of animals occurs all day, every day. When you watch undercover films of workers on factory farms or in slaughterhouses, you hear over and over again the workers roughly and angrily shouting at the terrified animals, calling them names that reference and degrade female sexuality: "bitch," "cunt," "whore," etc.

The parallels to the relationship between the sexes are undeniable. Some men frequently refer to women as "pussy," "bunny," "cow," "pig," and "chick" and to their body parts as choice cuts of meat: large hams and pieces of ass. A man may voice his preference in women by saying, "I'm a breast man" or "I'm a thigh man." Of course, the stereotypical female sex symbol, like the domesticated cow, turkey, or chicken, has to have excessively large breasts.

There is no doubt in my mind that the wearing of high heels by women is definitely a cultural aberration—symbolic of a culture accustomed to dismembering animals and hanging their parts in the butcher's window. When naked and walking on high heels, a human female, viewed from behind, bears a striking resemblance to the hindquarters of a cow, goat, or pig—animals whose hooves have the effect of elevating their rumps, making them look like they are walking on tiptoe. Advertisements for rib joints or barbecue restaurants often use images of pigs and cows wearing high heels and skimpy clothes.

The consumption of meat and dairy products, like the use of pornography, which degrades women, is a symptom of the disease of low self-esteem. Both activities result from the misguided notion that in order to feel sexier, younger, healthier, or stronger, one must exploit and consume the gifts of nature in any form that humans can readily dominate. In fact, the opposite is true. Long-term consumption of meat and dairy products can create any number of health problems, including heart disease, impotence, stroke, and cancer.

There is a higher incidence of impotence among meat eaters than vegans. A diet high in cholesterol is linked to sexual disorders.[55] The huge rise in the sales of pharmaceutical drugs used to increase sexual potency is evidence of our meat-eating culture's fear of losing virility. In India, milk drinking was, and still is, equated with male virility and the abundance of healthy sperm,

---

55 Fox News, "Is High Cholesterol Harming Your Sex Life?" Fox News (Aug. 13, 2008), https://www.foxnews.com/story/is-high-cholesterol-harming-your-sex-life.

but research has shown that drinking milk can clog the arteries and therefore increase a man's chances of developing erectile dysfunction.[56]

In modern times, eating meat and dairy products has been strongly linked to disease—not to health. Many diseases that have plagued human beings over the centuries stem from our mistreatment of animals. The stress of confinement suffered by enslaved animals brought about certain pathologies. With time, mutations allowed diseases to jump species: trichinosis and tuberculosis were originally diseases found in domesticated pigs, human influenza came from avian flu, horsepox mutated into smallpox, bovine rinderpest became measles,[57] and variant Creutzfeldt-Jakob disease is the human equivalent of mad cow disease.

In *The World Without Us*, Alan Weisman asks, "Could AIDS be the animals' final revenge? The human immunodeficiency virus that infects people is closely related to a simian strain that chimps carry without getting sick. Infection probably spread to humans through bush meat. On encountering the 4 percent of our genes that differ from the genes of our closest primate relations, the virus mutated lethally."[58]

Patanjali tells us very clearly that health and vitality will come to one who is established in brahmacharya— who treats sexuality with reverence. If we want to be healthy, we must consider the suffering, disease, and ill health we are causing to the animals we eat. Can we

56 "Impotence," Go Veg, https://www.goveg.com/impotence.asp.
57 Charles C. Mann. *1491: New Revelations of the Americas Before Columbus* (New York: Knopf, 2006), 98–99.
58 Alan Weisman, *The World Without Us* (New York: Dunne, 2007), 86.

really expect to be healthy by causing so much disease in the lives of others?

To embrace the practice of brahmacharya is to challenge our culture's foundation, which is dependent on the enslavement, domestication, sexual abuse, and exploitation of animals. When we talk about veganism and the practice of brahmacharya, we are definitely talking about a radical sexual revolution.

CHAPTER 7

APARIGRAHA

Greed, Excess, and Poverty

*Whatever joy there is in this world all comes from desiring
others to be happy, and whatever suffering there is in
this world all comes from desiring myself to be happy.*
—SHANTIDEVA, A GUIDE TO THE BODHISATTVA WAY OF LIFE

Aparigraha means "greedlessness." What happens when
one becomes established in greedlessness?

aparigraha-sthairye janma-kathantā-sambodhaḥ
PYS II.39
*When one becomes selfless and ceases to take more than
one needs, one obtains knowledge of why one was born.*

aparigraha: greedlessness
(**a:** not + **pari:** toward + **graha:** grasp)
sthairye: being settled or established in
janma: birth
kathanta: process of why and how
sambodhah: one has knowledge

WHEN WE DESIRE HAPPINESS FOR OURSELVES AT THE EXPENSE of others, it is called "greed." Patanjali recommends that yogis seeking enlightenment should try to live a simple life based in moderation rather than excessive consumption. In other words, "Live simply so that others may simply live." This is a radical concept to embrace these days, but yogis have always been radical.

Patanjali says that those who become established in *aparigraha* will come to know their future as they obtain knowledge of the processes that resulted in their birth. This is because practitioners come to a deep understanding that their birth, life, and imminent physical death, and the entire world they are experiencing is being created from their actions. The yogi begins to understand emptiness (*shunyata*)—how actions arise from one's perception of reality and how reality is never separate from one's perception of it. The yogi expands his perception of reality beyond the confines of linear time, dropping into a heightened state of awareness, which is the eternity of the present moment. This heightened state of awareness enables one to live more fully and more feelingly. As sensuality develops, empathy follows, lifting one out of self-centeredness into other-centeredness.

Through the practice of greedlessness, a yogi transcends linear time and is able to be free of wants. When we begin to contemplate the potential infinite results of our actions, we may begin to reflect on whether we can karmically afford certain actions.

Real needs are not wrong; wants, on the other hand, can become problematic. We are in the midst of a global crisis caused by insatiable human greed. The more we have, the more we want. Influenced by media imagery and advertising, we have become habituated to look outside of ourselves for happiness and, in the process, have created powerful addictions that drive our choices. Each time we allow an outside stimulus to program our actions, we allow our own inner power of discrimination to atrophy a bit, leading to further addiction. Many of us have become so out of touch with our innermost selves that we do not know where need ends and want begins. We become confused and use phrases like "I need to buy a new car" or "The kids need new school clothes" or "I really need you to do this for me" or "I need a drink," as if we would die without these things. We identify with what we have, need, and want. Due to *avidya* (ignorance), which gives rise to *asmita* (excessive identification with ego), we think we are our personalities, and with that thinking we lose touch with the true Self. The Self, which is whole and complete in its interconnectedness with all of existence, is sustained by love. One who identifies with this Self is a holy being, who knows when enough is enough and will never jeopardize the existence of the whole society for his or her wants.

A yogi practices self-reflection. This gives rise to *viveka* (discrimination), out of which arises wisdom, which leads to making choices that lead to enlightenment—not into deeper ignorance.

We have consumed far more than we need. The consequences for the survival of many animal species, as well as our own, are dire. The directive *aparigraha*, in contrast, helps one curb one's actions in accordance with what is good for all. Through aparigraha, we begin to understand ourselves as holy beings who thrive as part of a whole organism, working together for common benefit. We begin to feel our unique contribution to the wholeness of life. We come to understand that what we do is not small or insignificant to the lives of others or to the planet, but reverberates through every living being through time and space eternally. We become truly Self-conscious as we begin to realize ourselves as part of the greater whole of life and understand our destiny.

It is often argued that we alone possess self-consciousness and that all other animals do not and are only acting from an instinctual awareness, implying that they don't know why they are doing something or how their actions might affect themselves or others. For this reason, many people think that animals are a lower life-form and are less conscious and therefore undeserving of the same considerations we might extend to other human beings. I believe that animals are conscious. But, like us, some are more conscious of themselves and the world around them, and some are less so, and this can be influenced by age and illness. *Consciousness* means "joint mutual knowledge." The Oxford English Dictionary breaks the word down into *con* = "with, together" + *science* = "knowing of the whole" + *ness* = "exemplifying a quality or state." Thus, the word *self-consciousness* means "exemplifying the quality of knowing one's self as connected to the whole."

I have contemplated the assumption that animals are not conscious for many years while watching the way the deer and wild birds come to eat in our backyard in upstate New York. Never have I seen a deer or bird remain and eat all the food before moving on. A deer will come and take a few mouthfuls of grass, leaves, or seeds, lift her head and chew slowly, maybe lower her head and take another mouthful and repeat, and then walk away, allowing the next passing deer to sample some of the remaining food. I have never observed any wild animal staying and eating until there was no more food left. Nor have I ever seen any wild animal come with a bag or backpack, shovel in the food, fill the bag, and then carry it away so that there would be nothing left for others. No other animal besides us would destroy a whole forest or cause the extinction of an entire species while imagining that it has no negative effect on them or the lives of their future children.

Some people say that animals are less intelligent than we are because they don't make stuff. They don't build houses or shopping malls; print newspapers or magazines; manufacture rockets, airplanes, cars, or boats; or make plastic bags, televisions, cell phones, or computers. Perhaps animals have more developed intelligence and greater consciousness than we do, when measured by the ability to make connections. Many animals, because of their greedlessness, seem to have a deeper sense of how their actions might affect the greater whole. As they have managed to live without destroying their habitats, unlike us, perhaps many of the other animals are more conscious than we are.

If greedlessness leads to awareness, greed leads to denial. Many of us receive our first lesson in denial as children, when we question the morality of eating meat. As previously mentioned in the Prologue, when I was a child, I asked my mother, "If killing is wrong, isn't it wrong to eat animals?" My mother replied, "It's okay, because they are raised for that." This confused me even more. Another common response to that moral question is, "Yes, it is wrong, but it is a necessary evil." However, in his book *Dominion*, Matthew Scully responds with the question "When is evil ever *really necessary?*"

The German word *übel* means *evil*. The Oxford English Dictionary provides the same Germanic root for the word *über*, which means "up" or "over," meaning "to go beyond the limits of what is proper." In other words, that which is excessive is evil.

Earth provides enough to satisfy every man's need, but not every man's greed.

—MAHATMA GANDHI

According to the Food and Agriculture Organization of the United Nations, over fifty-two billion animals are killed for food worldwide every year.[59] If you visit the website Animal Rights: The Abolitionist Approach (www.abolistionistapproach.com), you can see the number of individual animals killed in the world every second. In the United States alone, approximately 10 billion land animals and billions of sea creatures are

---

59 Visit the Food and Agriculture Organization of the United Nations' Global Livestock Production and Health Atlas (GLiPHA) at http://www.fao.org/ag/againfo/home/en/news_archive/AGA_in_action/glipha.html.

slaughtered for food each year. It is hard to know how many sea creatures are killed because they are counted not as individuals but by tonnage. Regardless, any way you look at it, these are staggering numbers, especially if you consider that the human population of the United States is around 300 million, and that there are over 7 billion human beings on the entire planet. These billions of suffering and terrified animals create a planetary atmosphere of fear, terror, and violence, which we all live in and breathe every day.

One could easily call this amount of animal slaughter excessive. Farley Mowat writes in the book *Sea of Slaughter*, "The living world is dying in our time. . . . When our forebears commenced their exploitation of this continent they believed the animate resources of the New World were infinite and inexhaustible. The vulnerability of that living fabric—the intricacy and fragility of its all too finite parts—was beyond their comprehension. It can . . . be said in their defense that they were mostly ignorant of the inevitable consequences of their dreadful depredations. We who are alive today can claim no such exculpation for our biocidal actions and their dire consequences."[60]

We are devastating our oceans and emptying them of life. Many sea creatures are now extinct, and the number of threatened species is growing. Paul Watson, founder of the Sea Shepherd Conservation Society, says, "Seafood is simply a socially acceptable form of bush meat. We condemn Africans for hunting monkeys

---

60 Farley Mowat. *Sea of Slaughter* (Mechanicsburg, PA: Stackpole, 2004), 383.

and mammalian and bird species from the jungle, yet the developed world thinks nothing of hauling in magnificent wild creatures like swordfish, tuna, halibut, shark, and salmon for our meals. The fact is that the global slaughter of marine life is simply the largest massacre of wildlife on the planet."[61]

Human beings do not eat all the fish that is caught; most of it is force-fed to confined animals in factory farms to fatten them for slaughter. It may take 12–20 pounds of grain to make 1 pound of hamburger, but it also takes 100 pounds of fish to make that pound of hamburger.[62] Force-feeding animals like cows, who by nature are herbivores (vegans), the flesh of other animals—and sometimes even of their own species—could be deemed excessive and therefore evil.

Sea creatures suffer in other ways due to human greed. They starve to death because of lack of food. Their world is polluted by the toxic chemicals that we continuously flush into the ocean. Large fishing trawlers rake up many sea creatures that they did not intend to catch. The fishing industry refers to these beings as by-catch. When the hauls are sorted out, most of these creatures are either dead or dying and cannot survive the trauma of being caught, and they are thrown back into the ocean like so much garbage.

The relationship of humans to the Earth and all its creatures has been largely opportunistic, exploitative, and violent, resulting in a system of subjugation, domination,

---

61 *Veg News.* "The Veg News Interview: Captain Paul Watson." *Veg News,* March–April 2003: 25.
62 Ibid, 27.

and exploitation. We see the results of this all around us in the world today: pollution, slavery, war, division, nationalism, sexism, speciesism, and extinction. There is an alternative: Live so that your own life enhances, rather than impoverishes, the lives of others. This is not a new message. It is an ancient message with newfound meaning for the crisis we face today.

In my worldwide travels teaching yoga, I have found that human beings are pretty much the same all over; we are all looking for happiness. For the most part, the people I meet who are interested in yoga are dissatisfied with the present culture, which propagates the idea that happiness can be achieved only through material wealth gained through the exploitation of the Earth and other beings. The people I meet seem to want to break free from a commodity-driven way of life to find a new way of living that is more kind, simple, fulfilling, and selfless.

As His Holiness the Dalai Lama recommends, "Think of the problems in the whole world as your fault." To care for others is in our own self-interest. His Holiness calls this "enlightened self-interest." To dare to care about the happiness of others is to awaken the power of unconditional love within you.

---

te samādhāvupasargā vyutthāne siddhayaḥ PYS III.38
*By giving up the love of power, you
attain the power of love.*

---

te: they (referring to the *siddhis* or powers)
samadhav: for the attainment of enlightenment;
cosmic love
upasarga: obstacle
vyutthane: outward show
siddhayah: supernatural powers

Jimi Hendrix must have been channeling this yoga sutra. In any case, the message of love as the greatest power continues to ring true. The power of love cures the disease of low self-esteem, which is a pandemic in our world today. There are no "ordinary people"! Everyone is a manifestation of the Divine. Through the practice of yoga, people begin to remember this. They become Self-confident through a deep inner connection with the eternal Self, which is the real essence of every being. The nature of that inner Self is joy.

When one feels this joy and confidence, one is less likely to hurt others. The underlying reason we hurt others is our ignorance (*avidya*): We don't see the soul and divinity in other forms of life. This is at the core of the question of why human beings eat meat, enslave and exploit animals, and go to war with other people. If we felt Self-confident, we would not be inclined toward violence and greed. We would have a peaceful world free of poverty, slavery, and war.

Through the practices of yoga, we discover that concern for the happiness and well-being of others, including other animals, must be an essential part of our own quest for happiness and well-being. We realize that we can never be free as long as we participate in enslaving others. As our ability to be compassionate and extend our compassion to include animals grows, we heal the disease of disconnection so prevalent in our culture, and we begin to feel whole again.

We begin to see that it could be possible to create peace on Earth while living a liberated life—the life of the jivanmukta. Through adopting a compassionate, vegan way of eating, we take the first big step toward becoming established in aparigraha, and with that, we step into a bright, enlightened future for ourselves, for the animals, and for this planet.

Our culture has conditioned us over thousands of years to hoard, stockpile, accumulate, and save for a rainy day. The number of things we feel we own gives us a sense of security and creates a legacy of self-importance that we want to pass on to our children in the hopes of being remembered or immortalized. Buying power is a much sought-after *siddhi* in our modern times.

Shopping is a major part of most human lives. Much of what we work so hard to buy, we don't even really want. Soon, we get tired of it and throw it away, thus creating throwaway or disposable societies. I read that 85 percent of everything purchased in an American shopping mall ends up in a landfill within two weeks after purchase. Activist Julia Butterfly Hill asks, "Where is this place we call 'away'?" Of course, it doesn't exist. Each time we designate something as trash, we lose something of our own souls in the process. In the languages of many indigenous cultures, where there is perhaps more of a kinship felt with other animals and the Earth, there are no words for trash or garbage; the concept of throwing something away doesn't even exist.

Our consuming and hoarding behavior has been evolving for thousands of years. Early on, when we began to domesticate and enslave animals and to farm the land, we also developed methods to preserve the surplus of harvested food. We came to think of the flesh and milk of animals in the same way as the vegetables we plant, grow, harvest, and hoard—as wealth that enables us to market, buy, and sell. Over thousands of years, we have cultivated this way of life and the belief in the necessity of it. We instill in our children a certainty about the need to work and along with it the concept that work somehow differs from life itself.

We divide our lives into workdays and vacations, or days off. Many of us think of work as something we do to enable us to live but do not consider it something that we like or prefer doing. This is a strange idea, since during the many hours we spend working, we are also alive! Still, we often feel that our work is not what we really want to be doing, that it is only a means to an end, and that our real life begins after work.

We have created a relationship with time in which we believe that life is made up of a series of events, the causes of which are random, and the end result is a mystery. Civilized humans have lost their connection with the cycles of nature. We have become time-bound, enslaved to the clock and wristwatch. When we exist fully in the present moment, there is less fear of not having enough in the future and less inclination to greedily stockpile a surplus. Through the practice of aparigraha, the yogi becomes conscious of his or her true existence as having never been born and with that realization is able to defeat death. For it is only those who insist they were born who will die.

Yoga provides a door to the infinite through the experience of multidimensional reality. Eternity is happening now for the yogi who becomes unfettered by the conventional restraints of linear time. Such a yogi dismantles the ancient prison walls built by the bricks of greed and held together by the mortar of fear. All fears come down to the fear of losing: losing fame, youth, money, hair, health, love—but ultimately life. If one thinks of oneself as mortal, one's whole life will be haunted by the fear of death (abhinivesha), which, according to Patanjali, is a great hindrance to Yoga. To let go of the desire to possess is to be liberated from the fear of death.

When the yogi realizes the eternity of the Self, he or she becomes unbound by time and freed from the cycle of birth, life, and death. This new level of consciousness allows the imagination to explore the infinite possibilities of simultaneous existences. As one becomes unchained from linearity, the illusion of rational thought dissolves as intuition dawns. This dawning will be swift and timely as intuition envelops the parts into the whole to give birth to a brand-new day.

We are on the brink of an apocalypse that some have prophesied will result in a radical shift in how we relate to time. The Greek word apocalypse means "reveal; uncover; stand naked, exposed without artifice, clothing, or possessions." When we let go of holding on to things, our hands will be open to receive everything.

This *yuga*, or present age, has been spoken of in Hindu scripture as the *Kali Yuga*. *Kali* is derived from the Sanskrit word *kala*, meaning "time." Some say that beginning with the year 2012, a dawning has appeared, ushering in a new relationship to time as we have previously come to regard it as distinct from the infinite aspect of space, and with this dawning will come a bright awakening—a glorious revelation of new possibilities. A new age will be born. As with all births, it will be a bloody matter, but it will result in wondrous potential. Perhaps our true potential will be revealed to us as caring, nurturing beings who see ourselves as an essential part of a whole—who see ourselves as holy.

Certainly, we must all agree that our present greed-driven, consumer-based culture will not sustain the Earth or us, as it is destined to throw us all away. We must find a more harmonious and mutually beneficial way to live with all beings, where we distinguish between need and greed and act accordingly. Technological advancements are happening at an accelerating pace, but is our consciousness? Until we actually feel infinity, time will run out, and we will never experience a time/space continuum: a multidimensional place not bound by the past or future. It won't be too long now until time will be no longer, and death will be the last thing to die.

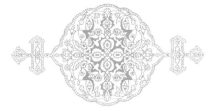

CHAPTER 8

LIVING THE LIFE OF A JIVANMUKTA

Spiritual Activism

*Never doubt that a small group of thoughtful,
committed citizens can change the world.
Indeed, it is the only thing that ever has.*
—Margaret Mead

*The greatest threat to our planet is the
belief that someone else will save it.*
—Robert Swan, environmentalist

Jiva means "individual soul" and *mukta* means "liberation." A *jivanmukta* is a liberated soul—one who knows himself or herself to be one with all that is. A jivanmukta is a living liberated being who works to contribute to the liberation of others.

If you look deeply into Patanjali's Yoga Sutras, you will find that in this ancient scripture, there is a direct reference to spiritual activism. It heads off the second chapter, the chapter that offers practical methods a person can do to attain Yoga, or at least come closer to it.

tapaḥ-svādhyāyeśvara-praṇidhānāni kriyā-yogaḥ
PYS ll.1

You must be fueled by a burning desire to work hard, continuously study the Self, and devote all of your efforts to God; these are the actions to be taken to attain Yoga.

tapa: heat, discipline, hard work
svadhyaya: study the Self
ishvara: one's own personal God
pranidhanani: offering one's life force to
kriya: purifying action
yoga: enlightenment, realization of the Self, reconnection to the eternal source, linking to God

This sutra speaks of the yoga of activism, which Patanjali refers to as Kriya Yoga. *Kriya* is a Sanskrit word meaning "purifying action." Yogis are interested in purifying themselves from the "dirt" of avidya, which refers to ignorance of one's Divine nature—who you really are, your true identity. Most of us who are unenlightened identify with our ego, our personality, our body/mind self. This misidentification causes us to think we are the doer, and with that, arrogance arises. An activist who thinks he or she is going to change the world through his or her own efforts is clouded by avidya. Activism motivated by the ego-self often resorts to aggressive, angry methods that usually end in frustration and disappointment for the activist and don't further the cause.

Patanjali offers another type of activism—a method of linking the actions of small self with the eternal Self, and thus becoming a channel for compassion, enabling one to work *with* rather than *against*. He offers this yoga of action as a three-step program involving commitment, discipline, and hard work; activism is not for the passive layabout. Spiritual activism demands enthusiasm—being enthused, divinely impassioned: Make time to study your true eternal nature, don't get caught up in your temporary body/mind existence and the dramas of your egoic personality, and devote your life, all your actions, to God and become an instrument for Divine Will, which means being the embodiment of unconditional love in the world. This is how lasting positive change can be implemented.

A spiritual activist is actively involved in shifting from an egoic sense of doership to being an instrument for a higher power. A spiritual activist is actively trying to let go of his or her identification with I-, me-, and mine-ness. Spiritual activists could be called yogis because they are interested in yoking to, connecting with, plugging into the spiritual source of being and channeling that energy. When this channel is activated, what can be accomplished on the material plane has infinite possibilities. Love awakens and activates the soul. God is Love. With great Love, all is possible. Love is the power that unites—dispelling separation, prejudice, and fear.

An activist is someone who actively works for change. To be spiritual is to feel your connection to all living beings. Spiritual activism is to actively work to further the conscious connection of oneself to others in a positive, life-affirming, mutually beneficial way. To be a spiritual activist is to be activated by spirit rather than a skin-encapsulated ego. To dare to care about the happiness, well-being, and liberation of others is to be a spiritual activist. A jivanmukta actively pursues liberation or enlightenment for the benefit of all.

The biggest obstacle to our spiritual evolution as a species at this time is our perception and treatment of animals and the natural world. Once we wake up from our sleep of denial and become aware of the truth of our connection to all of life, our *sadhana*, or spiritual practice, begins.

Philosopher Arthur Schopenhauer said, "All truth passes through three stages. First, it is ridiculed. Second, it is violently opposed. Third, it is accepted as being self-evident." After you are exposed to the truth of how animals are treated by today's agribusiness and how the members of our worldwide culture perpetuate this treatment through the meals they eat and products they buy, it will be difficult for you to continue to live the life you previously led. The most difficult thing for many people who become awakened to the reality of animal abuse is to figure out how they are going to help stop the abuse. Inaction is not an option for the yogi, but how to act in the most effective way may not be so obvious at first.

When people learn of the horrible animal abuse that goes on day after day, they typically react in one of two ways: Either they feel despairing, overwhelmed, and helpless, or they get angry and want to attack the perpetrators.

Neither one of these reactions will bring about a positive transformation that will benefit the animals. It will take intense passion of the best type: compassion. Only through active, conscious compassion can you affect people's minds and hearts, with the result that they find it in themselves to be compassionate and to extend that compassion to all beings, including animals. In other words, change must start with you; you must become the embodiment of compassion. You must treat the people you are speaking with in a compassionate manner, no matter how outraged you may feel. Even though you now know the facts about how animals are abused and how this is causing mass destruction of the planet as well as our spirits and our health, you must use yogic self-control and temper your passion with compassion. If you come across as preachy, angry, or judgmental, you most likely will not be able to hold an audience long enough for them to begin to hear the truth of what you are saying.

As you begin to speak of the truth you have experienced about how animals are treated, you will likely be ridiculed by others at first, even by friends and family members. Accept this as a natural phase in the process for people whose lifelong conditioned assumptions are being challenged. Hang in there, and stick with your principles. Patanjali suggests that when you find yourself in a difficult situation, turn it upside down. See it as an opportunity, not as an obstacle, and, most important, don't get angry.

---

vitarka-bādhane pratipakṣa-bhāvanam PYS II.33
When disturbed by disturbing thoughts,
think of the opposite.

---

vitarka: negative thought
badhane: to overcome; make beneficial
pratipaksha: the opposite
bhavanam: should be thought of

When destructive emotions like hate, anger, or the desire to do violence arise within you, cultivate the opposite state of mind. See the other person's potential for kindness and bolster your own expression of kindness. View others with hope, seeing them as having overcome their own ignorance. If you see them in a negative way, the power of your perception will only help to keep them that way as you polarize yourself from them, assuming a superior role.

The ridicule you may endure from others when you speak up for animals can help you hone your skills, enabling you to become better at articulating the message of veganism and animal rights in an informed and compassionate way.

As the others around you realize that your principles will not be easily shaken by their dismissive attitude, they may come to feel threatened. When people's lifelong habits and assumptions are threatened, they may display violent opposition to the truths you are helping them realize. When huge corporations feel financial threats to their profits, they will undoubtedly react with aggressive opposition. Remember: The key to the success of the animal-user industries has been the ignorance of the consumers and their unquestioned trust in authority.

As the stakes get higher, these industries and their long-standing governmental supporters will take drastic measures against those who act to support the liberation of animals from human exploitation. Hang in there. This is only phase two. Acceptance of truth is bound to come, because it is what underlies our ground of being. The truth is that we are one, appearing as many. How we treat each other will be reflected in the individual as well as in the whole. Many people, when they finally come to accept something as truth, will deny that they were ever in opposition to it. Fine; don't worry about that. Celebrate every step anyone takes toward becoming more conscious and more whole. The steps to truth are the steps to holiness.

The individual is capable of both great compassion and great indifference. Humans have it within their means to nourish the former and outgrow the latter. Nothing is more powerful than an individual acting out of conscience, thus helping to bring the collective consciousness to life.
—NORMAN COUSINS, JOURNALIST AND PEACE ACTIVIST

Now that you have an understanding of spiritual activism, the deeper meaning of asana, the kleshas and how they bind us with ignorance, arrogance, prejudices, and fear, and the yamas and how the way you treat others affects not only them but also what happens to you, you will be able to go beyond an intellectual grasp of these concepts provided by Patanjali. Through experimentation and reflection, you will come to experience the proof of these ideas through the daily experiences provided by your own life.

Others will undoubtedly ask you questions like "How and why do you practice yoga?" and "Why do you eat the way you do?" I hope the following advice will help you connect to that innate, compassionate part of yourself where your unique problem-solving skills lie, waiting to be expressed.

The real question is "How do you unearth and develop compassion within yourself so that it is what motivates your interactions with others?" Compassion is the essential tool if you want to be an effective speaker on the subject of yoga and veganism. If you have a desire to speak to people and help them understand why they should care about animals and adopt a vegan diet, these ideas may help you achieve your goals.

1. LISTENING: The Heart of Communication

First, be sure you *want* to communicate. Many people are concerned only with expressing themselves, which isn't necessarily communication. Communication implies communing, having a shared experience with another, not "talking at" someone. Merely professing what you know is not communicating. Listening is essential to communication, taking into consideration the person you are talking to and where he or she may be coming from. Through empathy, consider why people might be doing certain things you would like them to change. To develop empathy toward someone who is doing something you consider morally or ethically wrong, try to realize these facts:

1. Whenever people are doing anything, they are doing the best they can at that time.

2. When someone is doing something abusive, they are getting something that they feel is positive from the experience.

Through empathetic listening, you will be able to change underlying causes, not just outward symptoms. Nonviolent communication with others you would like to inspire toward change will transform you in the process, as it will develop compassion, which dissolves differences and leads to an enlightened existence.

If we, as yoga teachers and practitioners, are to communicate the radical ideas of yoga, we must address controversial topics such as animal rights and veganism. To do so successfully, we must focus our time, efforts, and skills to their greatest effect. It will serve no one if we get burned out, losing sleep over the fact that we haven't accomplished world peace, the end of war, and global veganism overnight. Instead, we can make real gains by focusing on specific real opportunities that surround us every day, such as the people who come through our doors seeking yoga, those who are asking us to teach them the means to become happy.

A yoga teacher aims to communicate rather than profess or preach. To communicate, one must be able to listen and to hear where the other is coming from. A yoga teacher must begin with an understanding of compassion as the ultimate cause of enlightenment. Whatever methods the teacher shares with the student should awaken compassion within the student—compassion not only for others but for themselves as well.

When we want to speak about yoga to someone who is still eating meat and does not see the karmic connections between what they are doing and their present physical, emotional, mental, or spiritual condition—or even their potential future condition—we must first find a way to communicate with them. It's no use condemning them. Instead we must listen in order to "hear" their present condition.

Eating meat and consuming milk products is an addiction: an addiction to violence. To facilitate a lasting positive change, we must view the person who is still eating these foods in the same light as we would view a drug or sex addict.

Rational arguments usually don't have much effect on addicts. Drug addicts, for example, may have an intellectual understanding of their problem, and may even say they want to stop, but they can't because of physiological and psychological addiction. A better approach to the issue would be to appeal to the heart of the addict. This takes skillful communication, starting with the ability to listen. One must be careful not to condemn violent acts through guilt. Guilt is not an effective way to initiate a lasting change of heart in an addict. We must go to the heart and help the person enter into a deeper feeling level of his or her own being and connection with all other beings. This is what a yoga teacher does.

We must probe deeper and try to understand the possible motives for the person's actions. When someone is engaged in a "bad" action, in his or her mind, the person believes he or she is getting something "good" from the action. If we want to try to help someone stop destructive actions, we have to look at the benefit the person thinks he or she is getting. We must view the person through the eyes of compassion. We must see the person as whole and complete and communicate to the person from that viewpoint, recognizing that his or her habit of causing harm to others is coming from a deep feeling of incompleteness within. We must address the *avidya*, or underlying lack of true Self-confidence and Self-esteem. To begin to do so, we must first find a way to communicate, which means listening to the suffering of that other person; this will awaken our compassion and provide us with the skills to take the necessary actions. We must discover the cause of this person's actions, not merely address or condemn the symptoms.

I recall an interview with psychologist Dr. Marshall Rosenberg in which he described his work with prisoners incarcerated for being child molesters. Rosenberg spoke about one particular prisoner who had shared his story after several sessions. As with many cases of child abuse, the prisoner himself had been abused as a child. When asked by the doctor to describe his childhood experience, the prisoner vividly described the horror and trauma he had gone through at that time. He also intimated that his experience had been all the more horrific because he could not communicate his fear and terror to anyone. Even when he had tried to communicate, he found that the other person could not understand what he was describing because the person had not been there and felt what he had felt.

Rosenberg then asked the obvious question: "If it was such a horrific experience for you, then why would you want to do this to other children?" The prisoner replied, "When I saw the fear and terror in the child's face, I knew, at last, that I was with someone who understood what I had gone through."[63]

Perhaps all the violence in the world today could be seen in essence as a failed attempt to communicate. True communication depends on not just one party expressing himself or herself, but on both parties listening to each other and developing a shared expression.

Through compassion, real communication is possible. If we, as activists, want to stop violence against animals, we must offer a clear, lasting, positive solution that will satisfy all parties. We can't just condemn and vent anger against meat eaters. This is an important point for the activist to remember. We must override the tendency within ourselves to perpetuate the good guys/bad guys, winner/loser, or victim/perpetrator syndrome. Our ultimate aim must be a win-win outcome for all: for the animals, the former animal exploiter, and even ourselves.

Yoga provides practical methods to communicate through developing one's ability to listen. Take, for instance, the yogic method of practicing asanas—

---

63 Marshall Rosenberg. *Speaking Peace: Connecting With Others Through Non-Violent Communication* (Boulder, CO: Sounds True, 2003).

especially twisting asanas. They address on a gut level the ego or separate-self and bring awareness to the organs of digestion and assimilation of food. This can awaken latent or buried feelings of anger, depression, or low self-esteem, which have been subtly held in those organs. Through practicing asanas, one can begin to unearth the causes of their destructive tendencies and heal the disconnection. People eat meat in an attempt to feel better about themselves—to feel healthier, sexier, stronger, or more empowered. They mistakenly feel that by taking the life of another, they will gain power. Instead, they become addicted to an illusion of power and are ultimately weakened, because their sense of power comes from disempowering another, not from the source of power itself, the Self, which resides within and whose nature is unconditional love.

This ignorance or mis-knowing is a case of mistaken identity and leads to deeper external and internal disconnection and further violence. And as the process is repeated over and over again, the person finds himself or herself caught in a net of debilitating addiction. The yoga student, through the practice of twisting asanas, becomes aware of his or her negative feelings and can begin exploring their root cause to find why these feelings exist, ultimately becoming more open to the message that perhaps eating meat is contributing to that negativity.

If you are to succeed in assisting others to overcome addictive and selfish behaviors, it will be due to compassionate communication, and if you succeed in pointing the way for others toward the liberating process of enlightenment, they will be able to reach it only through their own deep compassion. If you can convey this—if you can somehow graft compassion into the hearts of others by your example—you will have given them the greatest gift.

2. FEELING: The Means of Communication

IF YOU WANT TO TRULY COMMUNICATE TO OTHERS, THEN before you speak, ask yourself:

> How do I want them to feel about themselves when I talk to them?

One of the most inspiring speakers I know of is Dr. Martin Luther King Jr. I have studied his speeches for years, trying to glean a bit of what made him so effective, but it wasn't until I saw a documentary film about Malcolm X that I had an insight that gave me something new to consider regarding my own effectiveness as a speaker.

When Malcolm X spoke to African Americans, he addressed them as victims. He took every opportunity to remind them how they had been victimized by whites. He did this, I think, in order to move them to action. He wanted them to be angry about the way they were being treated so they would take justice into their own hands. He certainly had legitimate reasons to oppose the way blacks were being persecuted in America. However, I don't feel that he was effective in bringing about an enduring positive transformation, because he perceived himself and his audience as victims.

King had a different approach. He did not see African Americans as victims. He saw them as strong, whole, and complete. He didn't have time for hate, recognizing it as something that would slow him down on his way to his goal of racial equality. As he said, "I have decided to go with love. Hate is just too heavy a burden to bear." King envisioned a new world in which all people lived together in harmony, and he spoke from that elevated dream. Black people who heard him felt themselves to be strong, whole, and complete, empowered with vision and hope to take their rightful place in society rather than remain victims of an unjust racist system.

Only through humility and respect will you be effective in communicating. When conveying the messages of yoga and veganism to others, it is important you do not make them feel condemned or judged, but empowered to make conscious choices that would lead to liberation.

3. SEEING: The Expression of Communication

TO SEPARATE THE WORLD INTO GOOD GUYS AND BAD GUYS or victims and perpetrators will only result in more division, not the peaceful unification we seek as yogis. When you engage in conversation with others who may not agree with your point of view, be sure that you are coming from a place of tolerance yourself. King put it this way: "You have no moral grounding with someone who can feel your underlying contempt for them."

When you speak to others about veganism or animal rights, you must not view them as stupid, callous, or evil. Instead, see them through your eyes of compassion. See them as holy beings, capable of kindness. If the person eats meat, why not view that as a temporary condition? If you can't see others as potentially kind and compassionate beings, how can you ever expect them to see themselves that way?

We must remember that all beings—including the animals—find themselves in their present situations due to past karmas. This is not to say the animals deserve to be punished and we should condone or even contribute to their suffering. On the contrary, it is vital and essential that we do everything possible to alleviate the suffering of others. Our own liberation from suffering depends on it. To become spiritually activated is to feel the power of liberation operating within you. We must help the defenseless animal who is the victim of cruelty, and we must also extend our compassion to help liberate the human being who is the victim of his or her own blindness, which is the result of thousands of years of cultural conditioning. Only through compassion can real and lasting change take place.

When we accept that our karmas create our reality, we may awaken to a more compassionate understanding of the suffering of others. The law of karma is universal justice, designed not to punish, but rather to bring one to enlightened awareness through the empathetic understanding that arises through our past and present life experiences. The hunter driving a pickup truck sporting the bumper sticker "DEER ARE LIKE EGGS—THEY CAN BE POACHED" might reincarnate as the innocent lamb rescued by the farm sanctuary from the dead pile in back of a slaughterhouse. An abused animal may have been a meat eater a wink of an eye ago—we can't know for sure—but why not reduce our chances for reincarnating as cows and start drinking soy or almond milk? It's best, when interacting with anyone, to view all beings with compassion. The world certainly won't be any worse for it.

4. BLISS: The Result of Successful Communication

ECSTASY IS THE TRUE GROUND OF BEING, AND IT PULSATES within you at all times. Recognize it and celebrate it in others, and you will find it in yourself. By not trying to tame, enslave, and exploit others, you allow them the right to pursue their true natures and, in doing so, you allow yourself the same adventure into bliss.

If we are to spiritually evolve and survive as a species, we must liberate ourselves from the lie that we are separate from the rest of life. The world is a reflection of ourselves. By living in harmony with the Earth, we can find our way back to our true Self. I am not suggesting that we go "back to nature." That is not possible, because nature is with us now. It is who we are. Go within to experience the wildness of your own nature: that living place of harmony, where true anarchy—Self-rule—is the rule.

Establish your goals. Recognize the potential within yourself to become liberated and for your life to serve as an instrument of liberation for others. Cultivate your vision through infusing yourself with vast compassion that extends to include everyone.

How we treat others will determine how others treat us. How others treat us will determine how we see ourselves. How we see ourselves will determine who we are.

Never before in our known planetary history have we as individuals had such potential to decide our imminent future and that of this planet. If we are complacent and do nothing, the world as we know it will shut down. If, on the other hand, we come to our senses and dare to care about the suffering and happiness of others, we will abolish slavery in our lifetime and liberate ourselves in the process. *Moksha*, or liberation, is the goal of yoga, and ecstasy, or bliss, is its experience.

SPIRITUAL ACTIVATION

Angry thoughts disarray the heart
Pierce through the deformity with breath as your start
Shatter with a blow or a throw
You could do it inside a wishing well
Where your feelings once fell
If all else fails, embrace it with your holiness
Wrapping your everything around
Using the sound
Of the breath, what else could be better?
Yes that's it . . . the face of look upon you
Praying and Om-ing alone cannot do
Sitting at a lotus altar
While babies stumble to their slaughter
Nervous laughter holds you back from
Doing what you ought to
This Armageddon of look upon you

Is not going to stop, even in the forest, even in the shop
Hear the bodies going chop chop
It has only just begun
Birth is bloody—so many shades of red, she said
You don't know what it's like to be dead.
You heard them plotting to do disturbing things
What stopped you from intervening?
You are reeling in your obedience to ineffectualness.
Afraid of being humiliated? Stepping out of line?
Oh look at that face of look upon you!
Guilt paralyzes your mouth you cannot speak
Lies fill your ears, snuffing out the cries
Feet rooted in cement forgetfulness of who you are
So what to do?
Remember anyway and say something . . . anything
Pierce through the deformity
With a voice from the farm and the killing floor
When your own death is closing in
You will realize that the only thing
You ever really had in life was your effect upon others
Your end will come as a rattling snake slithering in
As you leave you will see that look upon you
You never ever had time, certainly no time to lose
Your body will stretch towards that last breath, so do your best
To see that all that you see is coming from inside of you
Nothing and no one has not been born from inside of you
Pierce through the deformity by means of breathing
Absorb into your rainbow body the pixilation of these phantoms
With the embrace of recognition
Allow black and white to collide into colors wondrous fair
And go on into the future of not knowing where.

CHAPTER 9

TRANSFORMATIONAL STORIES

The Life-Changing Power of Veganism:
Personal Accounts from Notable Vegans

IN RECENT YEARS, IT'S BECOME APPARENT THAT WE AS humans are radically questioning the way we see and treat other animals. Who would have thought that the rescue of a chubby rat stuck in a sewer manhole cover would have made front-page news worldwide? That's because it awakened empathy in us, even those who've historically hated rats and have fervently tried to anni-hilate the entire rodent species from the planet. (If you didn't catch this story, you should. The photo is pretty heartwarming.)[64]

When we hear about all the problems in the world today, from the devastation of the environment, global warming, water pollution, and wild-animal extinction to atrocious cruelties inflicted on farm animals, rising rates of cancer and heart disease to religious and

---

[64] Kathy Guillermo. "What Rats, Yes, Rats, Deserve: Why Did the Story of One Rodent's Rescue Captivate Us When So Many Humans Are So Thoughtlessly Cruel to These Animals?," *New York Daily News* (Feb. 28, 2009), https://www.nydailynews.com/opinion/ny-oped-sewer-rat-and-the-rats-in-our-lives-20190228-story.html.

political corruption and everything in between—health epidemics, mass murders, terrorist attacks, war, violence, and corrupt political and religious leaders—it's easy to feel helpless, and it may cause some of us to become cynical and angry, fall into blaming others, become depressed or suicidal, and give up.

But there is good news! These problems, on the other hand, have a way of motivating us to move in a better direction. Hope and optimism are the choices in front of us. This chapter features positive, inspirational stories from individuals whose lives have been transformed through the awakening of compassion.

KIP ANDERSEN

SAN FRANCISCO
Former cheese-aholic turned tofu-totaler . . .

Eleven years ago, as I was eating a cheese pizza, a twelve-minute PETA video narrated by Alec Baldwin, titled "Meet Your Meat," crossed my online path. Being a hardcore cheese-aholic, I sadly watched, for the first time, how dairy is made by using the breast milk from a mother cow whose baby was taken away from her, and other atrocities, such as how eggs are taken from hens and all male chicks are killed at birth because they can't lay eggs and are therefore redundant to the egg-laying industry.

As I watched the calf being taken away from her mother, I literally threw the pizza box across the room. I wanted the liquid sadness I'd just ingested to be cleared from every cell in my body as quickly as possible, and never to touch an animal product again. At the time, I didn't know a single vegan, and I was one of those people who thought there was no way to be healthy without animal products. Even though I really thought I may become anemic or die from deficiencies, I knew it was worth going vegan, as my life couldn't be so important that I had a right to cause so much harm to others. As I started doing research to learn more about what I'd seen in that video, I came across some facts about how raising and killing animals is also killing the environment! As I dug deeper, the connection between meat, dairy, and the environment only got worse—far worse. Reading study after study, I found that raising animals for food is the leading cause of species extinction, wildlife destruction, deforestation, water consumption, water contamination, ocean dead zones, and human-caused greenhouse gases. I was floored. How did I not know this? Why was no one talking about this? When I checked websites for my favorite nongovernmental organizations, no one was talking about it—the number-one destroyer of the environment—either. I felt let down and angry. I started reaching out to them but got essentially no response for months.

A bit more research revealed that eating animal products also contributes hugely to many health disabilities in the United States. It was mind-blowing. I didn't know much about karma then, but it all sure started to feel like it was making sense. The universe seemed to be shouting at us that this is what happens when we disrespect the Creator's creation.

At this time, I knew I had to do something more. I also knew it would be in the medium of film, as it is also a strong passion of mine. I didn't know how I was going to actualize it, other than that it simply had to be done. First, I started to look for others who were already speaking up about these issues to team up with. I wanted to connect with others who saw what was going on and lived accordingly to what they discovered. I figured this would be a good first step on the path to making a difference and sharing the Truth most effectively. This led me to yoga, as I figured everyone who practices yoga, since it is founded on ahimsa (non-harming), would be vegetarian or vegan. I figured that diving into a yogic practice would springboard me into alignment with my inner strength and make the vision of creating a powerful film come to fruition.

It was around the time that I realized not all yogis are vegan, or even vegetarian, that I discovered Sharon Gannon through an article in a yoga magazine, and learned of her book *Yoga and Vegetarianism*. I felt a huge sigh of conscious relief—here was someone who was making the connection between "us" and "others" and sharing that knowledge with the world. Soon after, I discovered Jivamukti Yoga and, in that, instantly found my tribe. I couldn't wait for the opportunity to take the teacher training so I could use it as a tool for activism, a tool to help me align with the proper vibrational way of being, with the strength and wisdom for creating a powerful film that would make a difference.

My dream of taking the Jivamukti Yoga teacher-training course came true in 2012. At that point, I'd already been trying to make my film for five years, and toward the end of the month of teacher training, I could finally see that my *trying* was transforming into *doing*. The charge, inspiration, and activation I got from all the tools I was developing were going to transfer into the actualization of this film.

I have countless happy memories from this time, but one of my favorites is when we had to write a pre-training essay about something we found important in yoga. I wrote that the most important asana practice is the one we do on our plates, and instead of using our arms and legs, we use forks and spoons (or in my case, chopsticks). Another fun memory that Sharon loves to share is that on graduation night, I humbly thanked her for all her work and for her voice for others and especially for courageously showing so many animal rights films in the yoga-training course. I expressed to her that I was there, at the training, to gather more tools to create "the film of all films" that will share the Truth with the world. My documentary would show what happens when we don't live in harmony with others as we were meant to, and what happens when we *do* live in harmony and respect all others as our brothers and sisters. She smiled at me and said, "Great—I can't wait to see it."

Eighteen months later, after gathering even more tools in India from a Kundalini teacher training with another of Sharon's good friends, Gurmukh, destiny introduced me to Keegan Kuhn, who would become my co-director/producer, and we introduced *Cowspiracy* to the world. As it turned out, it wasn't just the one film that had to be made. To combine all the elements of animals, environment, health, spirituality, and religion into one film was way too big a task, so *Cowspiracy* became a trilogy, along with *What the Health* and *Cowspiritual* (and then *Seaspiracy* and more films in the future). My promise to Sharon came true, and now my films are shown at all the Jivamukti Yoga teacher-training courses.

Sharon continues to be such an inspiration not just for me, but also for anyone who wants to speak up for the Truth and make a difference for those who need it most, whether they have two legs, four legs, no legs, or wings or gills, and especially for those that don't have a human voice at all. Mother Nature needs our voices, too, as not everyone can hear her screams and dreams; it is up to us to share them with her inhabitants. It is so wonderful to finally see a global shift toward the conscious realization that we truly are all One and that we have chosen to be on the right side of history.

KIP ANDERSEN is an American film producer and writer from San Francisco and studied at California Polytechnic State University, San Luis Obispo. He is best known for the film Cowspiracy: The Sustainability Secret. *Cowspiracy—a documentary co-directed by Keegan Kuhn and executive produced by Leonardo DiCaprio, became an overnight viral success and was followed by* What the Health *and* Cowspiritual. *He is a Jivamukti- and Kundalini-certified yoga teacher and the founder of AUM Films and Media, a nonprofit firm focused on creating movies that promote compassion and harmony for all life.*

MICHI KERN
MUNICH, GERMANY
From party animal and nightclub owner . . .

This is a story about inspiring and encouraging each other. This is a story about why doing good is the best way to live. This is a story about why yoga, for me, is 99 percent practice and 1 percent theory. This is a story about how being a radical vegan saved my life on two occasions. And this is my explanation for why "it's not over 'til it's over"—the most important message both in the Yoga Sutras and from the Rocky Balboa saga.

I opened Zerwirk, the first vegan restaurant in Germany, in 2004, in a sixteenth-century historical-landmark building in downtown Munich. The building had been used for centuries as a slaughterhouse and butcher shop specializing in selling parts of wild animals like deer and boar. After procuring it, I transformed its three floors into a vegan establishment, with a restaurant on the top floor, a concert space on the second floor, and a club on the ground floor. After about two years—and due to many noise complaints from the neighbors—we had to close the club on the ground floor, but we reopened it as a vegan deli, grocery, and retail store. The street where Zerwirk was located is called Ledererstrasse, which, in German, means "Leather Street," as it has many businesses that sell skins, bones, and flesh. For a while, sightseeing tours included "the vegan space" ironically located in the middle of a row of meat-based restaurants on their routes; there was a pork specialty restaurant next door that had a pig's-leg rotisserie in the window.

At the time, not many people in Germany had heard the word *vegan* or were familiar with the vegan lifestyle, so we met with a lot of opposition. Many people were afraid of us. Some of my close friends were even worried that I was going to *force* them to be vegan. It caused a lot of distress, but, I'll admit it was not bad as a marketing tool for a new restaurant!

On the night Zerwirk opened, Moby was in Munich playing a concert. We invited him to dinner at the restaurant before the show. He accepted the invitation and was our first guest, bringing along the whole tour crew. After dinner, he took me to the concert and announced from the stage, in front of thousands of people, the exciting news that a vegan restaurant had just opened in Munich. We received a lot of good press and rapidly became very popular.

But we had a major problem: There were no professional vegan chefs in Munich for us to hire! Our cook was an adorable hippie named Surdham Goeb, but he'd never cooked for more than four people in his apartment. Even so, he was committed to our vision. Surdham worked fourteen hours a day, and after half a year he was almost dead—not a very sustainable vegan lifestyle! After that, we hired a series of cooks, but unfortunately, the restaurant still lost too much money, and five years into the venture, my business partners and I closed our doors, exhausted.

Though it was disappointing, I believe the endeavor contributed to the visibility and popularity of veganism in our area. Now, there are more than ten vegan restaurants in Munich and the number is still growing, along with the number of vegans and vegetarians (now about 10 percent of the population). In 2017, my partner, Lissie Kieser, and I opened a vegan pop-up hotel, which immediately became *the place to be*. All along, we chose to employ Jivamukti Yoga teachers, because they were knowledgable and enthusiastic about spreading the vegan message and they walked their talk.

How has this evolution come about? I never stopped believing in the idea of ethical veganism and my partners and I never stopped promoting the idea with our various business projects, our personal lifestyles, and our teaching of yoga. Let me speak about David Life and Sharon Gannon, whose radical yogic teachings have inspired this evolution and revolution.

In 1999, I found myself with Sharon at the *Yoga Journal* Conference at the Fontainbleau Hilton Hotel in Miami Beach. We lined up at the buffet for dinner but found that there was nothing to eat for us vegans; even the green salad had cheese. As the only vegans there, we felt ridiculed by the other yoga practitioners around us, who thought we were just being picky. I was embarrassed, surprised, and angry. I asked Sharon, "What's wrong with these yoga people?" She smiled wisely and answered very calmly, "No need to get angry—they just don't have the awareness yet, but we are helping to change all that."

How did veganism save my life twice? I will tell you: I used to work for years as a club owner and doorman. Sometimes I would be harassed and bullied by rocker gangs at the door. One dark night after work, at about 3:30 in the morning, this one gang was verbally insulting me and taunting me for a fight. In the very last moment, the gang boss, looking like a raging bull, grabbed me and with his hugely muscled arm pulled my face next to his and said, "Listen, my friend, don't worry, we're not going to kill you. You saved my life, because I've been reading your Facebook postings and now I've become a vegetarian. Thank you! It's so cool—I feel so much better!"

The second way that veganism saved my life was that I met Lissie, who had worked for me as a server in my first vegan business in Munich. Now, we are raising two bright vegan children and live in a happy, cruelty-free vegan family. I am about to open a new vegan culture space as well as a second vegan pop-up hotel in Munich. In my spare time, I still teach Jivamukti Yoga, and I'm the co-director of the Jivamukti Yoga Center in Munich and the co-publisher of the German edition of the *Yoga Journal*. Not a bad outcome from all of this, reinforcing that good things do indeed come from doing good things. It is up to us to change the world one meal at a time and continue to share with others that the secret to happiness is to stop causing unhappiness to others. Veganism is the most simple and direct way to do that.

MICHI KERN *is a vegan father of two, restaurant entrepreneur, yoga teacher, publisher, author, and event producer with a bachelor's degree in philosophy from the University of Munich.*

INGRID NEWKIRK

SURREY, ENGLAND
Former police officer . . .

Imagine how odd it would be if you gradually stopped being a racist, one race at a time. Well, that's sort of the piecemeal way that I became a vegan.

At first, I stopped eating snails. That happened when I bought some—live—from an Italian market and, while driving the bag full of them home, noticed they had worked their way up to the neck of the bag. With their little tentacles and faces turned in my direction, they were staring up at me. It was disconcerting. The snails went off to find things to eat at the bottom of my garden, and all that delicious garlic and white wine I'd been planning to cook them in went down the hatch in other ways. No more escargot for me!

This was followed, months later, by what came to be known as the "lobster-dinner fiasco." It was a birthday celebration in a fancy Philadelphia restaurant. The lobsters came to the table on a silver tray, held by a waiter in a black tuxedo. I picked one. When that individual was brought back to the table, his back now split open and filled with butter and salt, I popped a forkful of his flesh into my mouth, anticipating the flavor. But it was not to be. Suddenly and most unexpectedly, from the depths of my subconscious, sprang a recollection: The lobsters had waggled their antennae at me as I made my choice. Could they have been trying to communicate in the only way they knew how that they were scared, that they sensed doom and didn't want to die? I had taken a living being and reduced him to a fleeting taste. A torrent of tears came out of nowhere. That was it for lobsters, crabs, and shrimp—and for the birthday dinner. No more crustaceans!

The end to my eating animals finally came when I was a deputy sheriff, dispatched to investigate a complaint about a farm in rural Maryland. The farmhouse door had blown open, and the wind had scattered the bills that had been pushed through the mail slot. Whoever had lived there had left in a hurry. Heading over to the barn, I could smell the corpses of abandoned animals who had starved to death—with the exception of one little resilient pig.

He drank water from my cupped hand, made little grateful grunting sounds, and let me pick him up and take him to my van. I completed my work and headed home. I was hungry and was looking forward to my dinner. What did I have in the fridge? I remembered that I had defrosted pork chops, and then the penny dropped. Wherever the pig those chops once belonged to had come from, I knew that his or her death had to have been wretched and frightening. No more mammals!

I didn't know any vegans then. I'm not sure the word had ever been spoken in the United States. There certainly weren't any foods marked "vegan" in the supermarkets or any soymilk at Starbucks. I hadn't a clue that there was any cruelty involved in that dollop of condensed milk that I poured into my tea every morning. That is, until one day a man saw me doing just that and asked me if I ate veal. Of course, I didn't. "But there might as well be a piece of veal in every bit of dairy you eat or drink," he said. "What?!" I replied. I listened to him as a child might look at a grown-up telling her there is no Santa Claus as he explained that there is no retirement home for a "dairy cow." That she is kicked and prodded down the same ramp those "beef cows" and pigs and lambs find themselves on. That a cow mother loves her babies with all her heart and that her calf is dragged away from her, often by one leg attached to a tractor pulley and often with her running behind the tractor, frantically crying out to him in desperation. All this so that the calf can be made into veal, leaving the milk that was meant for him to be stolen from her for my cup of tea. It was time to embrace black tea!

And so it was that I shed the chrysalis that had kept me from seeing the world as it is and emerged as a new vegan, anxious to explore. This exploration has brought me new flavors, new experiences, and new allies and, best of all, has stopped me from paying people to hurt and kill other living beings for my food. Having a clean plate is great—in more ways than one!

INGRID E. NEWKIRK is a British animal rights activist and president of People for the Ethical Treatment of Animals (PETA), the world's largest animal rights organization. She is the author of several books, including Making Kind Choices *(2005),* The PETA Practical Guide to Animal Rights: Simple Acts of Kindness to Help Animals in Trouble *(2009), and* Animalkind *(2020). Newkirk has worked for the animal-protection movement since 1972.*

VICTORIA MORAN

New York City

From Kansas City carnivore to Main Street vegan . . .

Dede was my first spiritual teacher. The grandmother-aged nanny who joined our family before my first birthday had studied the spiritual teaching of Rosicrucianism and Christian Science, and she'd visited mediums who could talk with the dead. When the nuns at school chastised me for suggesting reincarnation, Dede said, "They mean well; they just don't get out much."

One afternoon, I came home from first grade eager to recite the four food groups for Dede. These were the U.S. Department of Agriculture's dietary gold standard at the time, recommending that people eat daily from the meat group, the dairy group, the fruit and vegetable group, and the bread and cereals group. Dede responded, "Humph. There are people who never eat meat. They're called vegetarians. I could take you to a restaurant that serves hamburgers made out of peanuts and you'd think you were having beef."

We never went to the peanut-burger place, but hearing the word *vegetarian* awakened something in my soul; there it cavorted with my interests in mysticism and meditation and life after death, and a craving to know the meaning of it all. At seventeen, that desire led me to discover yoga—something that, in the 1960s, actually had to be discovered. I found three books on the subject in the public library and read each one over and over. They said that the first precept of yoga was *ahimsa*—nonviolence and reverence for life—and that if you intended to get serious about yoga, vegetarianism was not optional.

Shortly after high school, I moved to London for a fashion course. Amid that great city's vegetarian restaurants, well-stocked health food shops, and yoga classes, going vegetarian wasn't hard. Going vegan would be.

Even though veganism, as a philosophy and practice with a name and definition, was born in London, I didn't hear about it until I'd returned to the States. There, I connected with other vegetarians in a theosophical study group. Although decades older than me, these were my people, the ones I came to excitedly when I learned that you could be a "pure" vegetarian, a *vegan*. Their response was cautionary: "That's very extreme, dear." "Where would you get your calcium?" "Even the yogis use milk and ghee." I respected these elders—I mean, they were theosophists in Missouri—but I knew that vegans had the moral high ground. If consuming eggs and dairy meant that even one baby boy chick was macerated just after hatching, or one cow and newborn calf were forever torn from one another, it would have been wrong. Still, these atrocities were being perpetrated by the millions every single day.

So, I set about becoming vegan. I'd last weeks or months and then succumb to the convenient and the familiar. I was also dealing with a binge-eating disorder that had begun in childhood and progressed markedly in adolescence. It was discouraging to stand in a convenience store late at night, reading labels. It seemed that whey or milk powder or egg albumin made their way into every cellophane-wrapped temptation, so I'd give up, toss a few packets of cookies and snack cakes into my basket, and really stock up on my edible drugs of choice: cheese and ice cream. I was on and off with veganism—and yoga and happiness and peace—for almost twelve years.

During this period, I went for a bachelor's degree in comparative religions and earned a fellowship to undertake independent study on any relevant topic as long as I left North America to do it. I chose to return to the United Kingdom and explore veganism from a spiritual perspective in the country where the movement had begun. In today's dynamic vegan milieu, it's hard to imagine a time when there were so few plant eaters in the United States and Canada that an institution of higher learning would fund foreign travel to learn about them, but this was forty years ago, and that's the way it was.

Eventually, I entered a twelve-step recovery program for overeating. My sponsor told me that there are two kinds of spirituality: one you read about and contemplate and discuss, and the other you grab onto as if it were a life preserver. I needed that one. If I were ever to be free, the yoga principles I'd learned about and the religious teachings I'd studied in school had to become the way I lived my life, every day, every meal. That included consistently kind food choices, one day at a time. (Serendipitously, this happened just before my infant daughter started on solid food. Now an adult, she can claim lifelong vegan status, and she's built enough plant-powered muscle that she works as an aerialist and stunt performer.)

In 1985, the paper I'd written for the fellowship was published as a book, *Compassion: The Ultimate Ethic.* I never thought I'd write a book. Authors were people like Dickens and Tolstoy. Well, they're people like me, too, and the book I'm working on currently, about food and the soul, will be number fourteen. I've been fortunate to have written about and otherwise worked in the combined fields of spirituality, well-being, and veganism for over thirty years.

While I didn't set out to follow the traditional yogic life plan of student, householder, spiritual seeker, and renunciate, I see hints of it playing out. First, I had to be a student of life and spirituality in order to save myself from myself and live the *ahimsa* ethic. Then, I needed to raise my vegan daughter, work in the world, play with matter, and be fully present to the incredible gift of a life on Earth.

My third stage looks a lot like the second, but the motivation is different. I write, host the weekly podcast *Main Street Vegan*, travel, speak, and head up the Main Street Vegan Academy, an in-person program in New York City that trains and certifies vegan-lifestyle coaches and educators. That's hardly the life of a wandering ascetic, but what propels me every day is a spiritual prompting: the vision of a vegan world.

There is a fourth phase: detachment from material concerns and dependence solely on God. I don't expect ever to get that holy. Still, I like to imagine life at the completion of the mission: The world reaches vegan critical mass in time to turn around climate change and all people come to see that, in the words of the Jain saint Mahavira, "To every creature, his own life is very dear." After that, I may be inclined to focus quietly on matters of spirit, maybe locating those three books that introduced me to yoga so long ago and reading them, yet again, over and over.

VICTORIA MORAN *is the author of books including* Main Street Vegan, The Love-Powered Diet, *and* Creating a Charmed Life. *She is a speaker, podcaster, director of the Main Street Vegan Academy, and the producer of Thomas Jackson's film* A Prayer for Compassion, *which introduces vegan living to people of faith.* www.mainstreeetvegan.net.

RIMA RABBATH

BEIRUT, LEBANON

Former corporate marketing executive clicks the switch . . .

"Click!" The sound you hear when you press a switch. "Click" is a short sound. "Click" is the sound you hear when you turn the lights on. When I was a kid, I always wanted to keep the lights on. I never wanted to turn the lights off. Growing up in Beirut during the Lebanese Civil War (1975–1990), we were so often in the dark. The daily power cuts and blackouts would leave the entire city in total darkness for hours on end. So, whenever I had the opportunity to press a switch and turn the lights on, I would—and I would relish that short, quick sound, "click."

It was only years later, once I'd discovered yoga, that I realized the yearning to turn the lights on was symbolic of possibility—the possibility to see that which was surrounding me and to appreciate life, even if in its imperfect situation. It was the chance to see more than a foot ahead of me and to move around without feeling restricted.

The opportunity to move from Beirut to Paris for college came about when I was seventeen. After that, another move presented itself to me: America! I attended the New York University Stern School of Business. From there, I graduated with an MBA and joined Colgate-Palmolive in its marketing and brand management division, where I moved up the corporate ladder for eight years. It is during that time that I discovered the Jivamukti Yoga School on Lafayette Street in Manhattan and met my teacher, the extraordinary Sharon Gannon.

It is during that time that I understood my longing to turn the lights on as a kid was rooted in a desire to open my eyes wider. It wasn't just about turning on the lights, but about seeing my situation more clearly—*our* situation, whatever it may be, a situation that is deeply connected to the circumstances in which other living beings find themselves. Turning on the lights was the expression of a longing—the deep wish not to remain in the dark but to see the world with tenderness and sensitivity, and to stop ignoring the suffering of others, who are all, in essence, very much like me.

The awareness of how interconnected we all are with the whole of life is now integrated into my lifestyle. It's the invitation to live in such a way that prompted me to switch paths from my corporate career and teach yoga full time. As a Jivamukti Yoga practitioner for the past nineteen years and a teacher of the method since 2005, I have been inspired to find the connection. For example, the choices we make with our diet have the power to weaken or to strengthen the meat and dairy industries, which, combined, is one of the major blind spots of our economic system and a force that pushes us to look the other way so as not to see what is going on in our world. Looking the other way allows, and even encourages, behavior that is unconscionable, like the secret killing of millions of animals, who are kept in the dark until the "switch" of their slaughter, never to experience the beauty of daylight.

Ignorance, from the yogic point of view, is darkness. Ignorance is to bring down the shutters, to avoid the conversation, to choose not to see the suffering that takes place in the world, behind the shutters of laboratories that test on animals and factory farms where animals are separated from their mothers and held in cages, where animals cannot see more than a few inches ahead of them, where moving around is not possible.

So, a while back, I realized that this is not a story I want to be part of. Instead, I want to be part of a story of open shutters that let the light in, a story where my eyes are wide open because a light bulb went off and I've heard that "click," a story where I am able to see our precious world with clarity, for the goal of all yoga practices is to remove the veils of illusion and denial.

The story of living with awareness and eating with kindness is one we can all partake in. It is the story of our evolution and one that can never be put aside.

RIMA RABBATH is a former marketing executive at Colgate-Palmolive who is one of the most influential yoga teachers in New York. She has been teaching at the Jivamukti Yoga New York City School and leading the method's teacher trainings around the world for over a decade. She is known for her exceptionally curated music and her ability to reach a wide spectrum of students, encouraging people to start where they are and to use their practice and life as a journey of transformation.

MANIZEH RIMER

KARACHI, PAKISTAN

From an overworked techie surviving on coffee, bagels, and cream cheese . . .

In Karachi, at my Parsi grandmother's house, food was at the center of everything. My grandmother, Mahkusheed, and her three sisters, Ferengese, Parveen, and Bhaktaver (talk about unusual names), all lived next to each other in the same compound in Clifton. Some of my best memories were sitting around her table with my family, maybe up to twenty of us at a time, eating the most delicious, spicy dishes and feeling the joy of being together.

My mother was also an excellent cook; we always had fresh, home-cooked meals. My friends never missed the chance to come to my house for dinner. When I arrived at college in America, I put on 25 pounds during my freshman year—and I am petite! (I think this is called the Freshman 25.) I was introduced to the standard American diet (SAD) for the first time.

It was full of processed food. I was also eating so much more meat and dairy than I had ever eaten before. I panicked, ate less, cut out the free daily ice cream in the cafeteria, and lost the weight. Throughout my adult life, I never questioned *what* I was eating, as long as it wasn't making me put on too much weight.

That all changed in 2003. After years of working way too many late nights in the tech world, alternating between chugging coffee and NyQuil, my husband and I moved to London. I threw in the tech towel and went to the Jivamukti Yoga teacher training taught by the founders of the method, Sharon Gannon and David Life.

At that point, I still had no idea that what you ate had anything to do with Yoga. I remember being in total shock when it dawned on me that I had essentially been blind, or perhaps subconsciously ignoring the way we treat animals and how food was getting on my plate. In fact, when my husband came to visit me that weekend at the Jivamukti Yoga teacher training, he was waiting for me in a car parked outside the building. I emerged sobbing, just having watched *The Animals Film*, a British feature-length documentary and one of the first graphic animal rights films to be made. I was so upset after the film that I got in the car and could not talk. My husband thought I was being beaten with a stick by my newfound gurus! Far from it. In true guru fashion, all they had done was remove the muck from my eyes. I was also a little upset that I was no longer going to be able to live in blissful ignorance—it would have been so much easier!

I went on to open Jivamukti Yoga London and spent many years teaching at the center—my first baby. Then I went on to have two actual, human babies.

Many years later, my husband and I ended up moving back to San Francisco. I decided I wanted to extend my yoga practice from teaching to also investing—sounds like a paradox, I know. But investing in food startups that are providing vegan meat-replacement products to people is a natural extension of my yoga teaching. I created the Jivan Fund with my partner to do just that. The Jivan Fund supports projects such as the 2018 documentary film *Eating Animals*, based on the bestselling book by Jonathan Safran Foer, narrated and co-produced by Natalie Portman, and co-executive produced by Twitter co-founder Biz Stone. Beyond Meat, Good Eggs, and Amy's Drive Thru are all companies we back because we believe in them and think they are the future of food.

In 2003, when Sharon and David used to talk about veganism and yoga in class, people would walk out of the room. All these years later, talking about veganism to a room full of yoga practitioners is redundant. That's what I call progress!

MANIZEH RIMER *has a bachelor's degree in political science from Brown University. She is the founder of Jivamukti Yoga London and is founding principal of the Jivan Fund LLC, supporting startup companies that are doing all they can to make this world a kinder place for all.*

YELIZ UTKU KONCA, PHD
ISTANBUL, TURKEY
Former vivisectionist becomes a vegan scientist . . .

I discovered Jivamukti Yoga when I was a PhD student at New York University. Although I was living in the city of my dreams, doing the scientific research I'd been fantasizing about, and seemed successful by outside standards, I was feeling empty inside. I decided to give yoga a try and started to attend classes at the Jivamukti Yoga School.

The rigorous classes, complete with chanting, pranayama, and meditation, as well as philosophy and its application in our modern daily lives, helped transform my attitude toward life and instantly filled the emptiness I had been feeling. About a year later, in 2007, I took a sabbatical and enrolled in the one-month residential Jivamukti Yoga teacher training course. That experience was to change my life.

The assigned readings, the spiritual teachings, the philosophy, and the asana classes, along with the animal rights documentary films, were intense and compelling, causing me to deeply question many aspects of my life. During one particular class, I glimpsed a bird's-eye view of my scientific research and I burst into unstoppable tears. I cried for all the microscopic worms I was dissecting in the name of research, and for myself, because I was so blind to their suffering. That evening, I approached Sharon and David for advice. "Only you know what to do," they told me. "You have the solution inside of you." They continued to give this powerful reminder throughout the teaching; it echoed in my ears then and has been my guiding light ever since.

After the training, it was shocking to go back to daily life in New York City. The extent of animal abuse we were used to in our daily lives (in food, research, entertainment, and more) was now appalling to me. I had experimented with veganism before but wasn't able to completely make the switch. Then, one day, as I was taking a Jivamukti Yoga class and the teacher was talking about speciesism, I felt very vividly the similarity of a mother cow and a mother human. The love they both had for their babies was the same, their mother-baby relationship was precious, and I knew that nobody had the right to go between a mother and her child. I knew that I could no longer drink the milk of a cow if I wanted to live with integrity. I had to become vegan. I was terrified, and thought that I would become so sick and hungry that I would die, but it turns out I didn't!

After becoming vegan, I pulled away from the research that required dissecting microscopic *C. elegans* worms. I continued designing and synthesizing thera-peutic molecules, but I also started adding food-related analysis to my research profile. I worked with famous chefs in the research kitchen of the French Culinary Institute (now the International Culinary Center). I also participated in the founding of the Experimental Cuisine Collective, which brought together chefs, scientists, journalists, and farmers in monthly meetings.

I was now looking at everything from a vegan, sus-tainable point of view. At one point, we were working on an ice cream native to Turkey, which used a local wild orchid tuber that was going extinct. We were trying to save the orchid tubers by replacing them with sustainable sources, so why not also replace the traditionally used goat milk with sustainable plant-based milks? When the chefs used gelatin to clarify their chocolate sauces, I was suggesting plant-based alternatives that could give the same result. This thinking probably had an effect on my adviser at the time, who later became a member of the scientific advisory board for Beyond Meat.

Jivamukti Yoga taught me that caring makes a difference and that all of our actions have results. I started to see the advantage of being a scientist: I had the education to critically read and interpret scientific publications on vegan nutrition. So read I did.

Over the years, I've lived in New York, the San Francisco Bay Area, Los Angeles, France, and eventually Turkey, and had the chance to do research at many of the top research institutions around the world, including Caltech, New York University, NYU's School of Medicine, Columbia University's Vagelos College of Physicians and Surgeons, the Lawrence Berkeley National Laboratory, and Koç University in Istanbul. Most of my friends were scientists, and they asked me rational questions, and I felt obliged to find honest and scientifically backed answers for them. It was surprising to see, though, that even scientists, those rational, curious, objective people, did not acknowledge that the world is in crisis. Furthermore, those who did believed they could do nothing about it personally and were confident that science would eventually find an ingenious solution. They used the same denial methods that everyone else used in an attempt to stay in their comfort zone, deferring the responsibility to "science." Unfortunately, so many scientists still work to mitigate only the symptoms, rather than going to the root of the problem. I now teach chemistry at Koç University, where I try to teach my students to identify the root cause of a problem before they design solutions and to be aware of the consequences of their actions.

As a yoga teacher in Istanbul, struck by the lack of information on both yoga and veganism in Turkey, I decided to have Sharon's *Yoga and Vegetarianism* book translated into Turkish. Depressingly, I couldn't find anyone who wanted to make the effort to translate it, and no publisher was interested in publishing it. "It wouldn't be popular, and it wouldn't sell," they said. So, I translated the book myself and was able to find a publisher at the last minute. The book has been changing the lives of hundreds of yogis in Turkey ever since.

My knowledge of and expertise on vegan nutrition and how to adapt it to any condition or geography was put to the test by my two vegan pregnancies. Being a pregnant vegan scientist and yogi was the ultimate education. After completing two healthy pregnancies as a vegan (one in the United States and one in Turkey), I started to share my knowledge on vegan nutrition. Today, I am trying to educate as many people as I can through blog posts, podcasts, and trainings on sustainable vegan living.

Sharon had signed my copy of *Yoga and Vegetarianism* with the words "Thank you for daring to care," and today I can see the significance of being courageous enough to care about the happiness and liberation of all beings—human and animal. A bit more care and a bit more courage is all we need to transform our lives and the lives around us. It will help stop the destruction of the planet and all the beings who live here. As Sharon says, "Don't wait for a better world—start now to make it happen."

YELIZ UTKU KONCA was born in Bulgaria and educated in three countries: Bulgaria, Turkey, and the United States. She's a biological chemist by training who has been inspired by and trained in the Jivamukti Yoga method, which reminds her daily to be the one she's been waiting for. She's an 800-hour-certified Jivamukti Yoga teacher and has translated Yoga and Vegetarianism *and* Jivamukti Yoga *into Turkish. She lives in Istanbul, where she teaches yoga and vegan nutrition and is a university faculty member.*

BETH WATSON
WASHINGTON, D.C.
Former lobbyist for the U.S. pork industry . . .

I walked into my office, which was a stone's throw away from the U.S. Capitol, for an urgent, all-hands-on-deck meeting. The conference room was full of familiar faces: fifteen to twenty representatives from the meat and dairy industries. We were all there to confront a serious threat to the $800 billion–dollar meat industry. This threat wasn't a trade war, a product recall, or a deadly disease—it was a movie.

Earthlings, which was narrated by Joaquin Phoenix and portrayed a grim view of animal agriculture, was about to be released. The ad hoc coalition hired a Washington, D.C., public relations firm to refine messaging, place op-eds, and respond to an anticipated backlash against animal-handling practices—including potential legislation or state ballot initiatives. The coalition was preparing for a battle of hearts and minds, and nothing less than the "sustainability" of animal agriculture was at stake.

After doing their research, the paid consultants advised all coalition members to stay quiet. The film wasn't expected to have a large reach, and any attempt to combat its assertions would only draw more undesired attention.

A little bit about me: Following my college graduation, I was hired to conduct research and analysis on U.S. pork exports for an organization representing American pig farmers. Almost immediately, I stepped into a lobbyist role and spent my days developing relationships with House and Senate offices, building coalitions of like-minded organizations, and educating leaders on the importance of trade to U.S. agricultural communities—specifically, pork producers. I traveled with my colleagues every year to visit hog-farm operations, breeding facilities, and even slaughterhouses.

Generally, those of us in the animal-agriculture industry did very little to engage with congressional offices or organizations that vehemently opposed eating animals or were in favor of more restrictions on animal-handling practices. These "opponents" were seen as unreasonable proponents of veganism—an extreme lifestyle that, to us, indicated they were completely out of touch with reality.

It's been ten years since I left both the pork industry and the political world. I've also been vegan for over six years. When asked about my reasons behind this lifestyle change, I like to answer that I'm vegan for *all* the reasons (environmental, ethical, health-related, etc.), but I'm especially vegan for the animals. Everyone inevitably grows and changes over their lifetime, but I sometimes chuckle over my dramatic transition from a meat lobbyist to vegan yogi—how did that happen?

My story is not a heroine's tale. I didn't have a sudden change of heart before throwing myself in front of a pig awaiting slaughter. My transition was actually quite the opposite. It was a gradual shift that included a long period of physical, emotional, and intellectual opening. Though incredibly social in my mid-twenties, I was resistant to develop any real, loving relationships. After several years of trying to think my way through this emotional blockage, I decided to approach the problem *physically*. I started doing more back bends—both literally and metaphorically. To elaborate, I had been attending yoga classes at my gym and had begun frequenting a yoga studio in my neighborhood. Because the back bending had always scared me, I felt this wild urge to do more of it. For two years, I slowly developed a daily home yoga practice inspired by sequences that I learned online and in class.

During this same time, my life completely crumbled. My professional ambitions halted abruptly when I lost my job, and my family experienced back-to-back health crises. One day, I was a respected lobbyist wearing Jimmy Choos, toasting champagne at power lunches, and jetting off wherever I wanted; the next, I was unemployed and living at my parents' home in rural Minnesota as a caregiver for my mother and my grandmother. During those long, cold nights in northern Minnesota, I was forced to learn to sit and hold paradox. Though it wasn't necessarily obvious to me at the time, when the treasured ambitions that I'd pursued relentlessly over the years crumbled and I felt like my life was falling apart, my perceptions about what was truly important in life were also shifting. I softened and became a much more generous person—both to others and to myself.

After Christmas of 2012, I moved back to D.C. to look for work and get back on my feet. For our New Year's resolution, my husband and I decided to try a thirty-day vegan challenge (inspired by Jay-Z and Beyoncé), and I started attending yoga classes at a local Jivamukti-affiliated studio. When I learned that the studio was going to host a vinyasa yoga teacher training, I signed up without hesitation, as I felt desperate for wisdom teachings. Sharon Gannon's book *Yoga and Vegetarianism* was required reading for the course, and I was intrigued by her interpretation of the yamas. The idea that I could personally benefit from practicing kindness to others truly blew my mind. I eventually also found digital recordings of Sharon giving related teachings on the Jivamukti website; I listened to these on repeat for several months.

Within this same period of time, I finally watched *Earthlings* and was truly shattered by witnessing the suffering of animals for human consumption. It was that film that ignited my commitment to veganism—a commitment that included my pursuit of employment that would not have a detrimental impact on the lives of any creature.

This decision was a huge life shift—but this shift has not stopped. Interestingly enough, I have a deepening love for my former colleagues and friends who work in industrial animal agriculture. They are smart, kind, and reasonable people who are doing what they believe to be best for their families and the animals in their care. What changed in me was not a rejection of rational thinking, but rather the cultivation of a desire to identify the root cause of suffering. This ongoing journey of mine has completely changed my understanding of how we relate to ourselves, fellow humans, animals, and the Earth.

As a new mother, I've come to learn that the constant misrepresentations of farm animals begins very early on in life. For instance, many children's books and story rhymes portray farm animals as happily rolling in the mud or playing in the hills with their "friends." These idyllic scenes do not accurately represent the daily lives of most animals that are raised for human consumption. Because of this realization, I hope to instill kindness and compassion for all living beings in my daughter—and perhaps one day she will choose to remain vegan.

BETH WATSON *is a Jivamukti Yoga teacher and a user-experience and organizational-design consultant living in Washington, D.C. She helps teams envision a better world and commit to the essential practices to see it through.*

CHAPTER 10

GETTING STARTED ON A VEGAN DIET

21-Day Cleansing Diet

MANY DOCTORS AGREE THAT IT TAKES ABOUT THREE weeks (twenty-one days) for the human digestive system to rid itself of toxins and to free us from destructive eating habits and biochemical addictions.

Meat and dairy eating is addictive. How is this possible? Neal Barnard, MD, explains in his book *Breaking the Food Seduction*: "Scientific tests suggest that meat may have subtle drug-like qualities. . . . As meat touches your tongue opiates are released in the brain. . . . Meat stimulates a surprisingly strong release of insulin. . . . In turn, insulin is involved in the release of dopamine between brain cells. Dopamine . . . is the ultimate feel-good chemical turned on by every single drug of abuse—opiates, nicotine, cocaine, alcohol, amphetamines, and everything else."[65] Barnard makes a similar point about cheese.

First, viewing yourself with compassion is essential for the success of any diet program. Guilt-tripping and negative projection are never helpful. If you can free yourself from your destructive addictions, you will discover

---

65 Barnard, *Breaking the Food Seduction*, 63–64.

that within your own body is a pharmaceutical laboratory that can provide you with the well-being you seek. But to become independent, you must first give yourself the chance of experiencing your body when it is not hampered by addiction so you can begin to feel its innate intelligence. You may feel that going from the standard American diet (SAD) of meat and dairy products to a 100 percent organic vegan diet overnight may be too much. Or maybe your schedule is too busy to allow you to stay on it for the full twenty-one days. The important thing is not to beat yourself up and feel pressured to change overnight. Instead, just try this diet for one day without feeling you have to commit to a vegan diet for the whole rest of your life. Even eating vegan for one day will be greatly appreciated by your body and mind and by the animals, as well as the greater world we all share.

But if you are up for the full adventure, follow this simple diet for twenty-one days to give your digestive organs a rest and gently help them transition to a healthier diet. This diet will reset your metabolism and help free you from biochemical addictions triggered by food, drugs, and emotions.

This is by no means a starvation diet; it provides ample food and lots of fiber. You will find that you are not hungry, nor will you have problems with constipation. This diet is vegan, eliminating all animal-based foods. In addition, it does not include wheat and soy, because sometimes these foods cause allergic reactions. Oil is eliminated as well, to help you lose unwanted weight and give your gall bladder and your liver a rest from the job of metabolizing fat. Drugs, alcohol, and caffeine are eliminated to help clear the thinking mind and allow you to reflect on how you deal with stress. The elimination of drugs, alcohol, and caffeine also provides your nervous system and internal organs—especially the liver and the kidneys—a rest from having to process these challenging substances.

Salt and sugar are taken in minimal amounts. You will get some salt from the seaweed in the nightly kitchari soup (see recipe on page 197), and you will get some natural sugar in the fruit and juice. Eliminating salt will help release fluids from your tissues and reduce swelling and puffiness. Many times, when we feel we look "fat," it is not fat we are seeing but water retention. Eliminating sugar helps the overall metabolism become more balanced and stable and less prone to cravings and binges.

As the food you will eat will be blended or porridge-like, it will aid in digestion and give your jaw a rest.

Make sure that all you do choose to eat is organic so as to minimize adding any new toxins to your own bodily system or into the greater system we all share: the Earth.

You will eat two meals a day—oatmeal for breakfast and a porridge-like soup and blended salad for dinner—with a lunch snack.

Here is a list of the staple food items you will need to have on hand:

- Old-fashioned oatmeal (not instant or prepackaged)
- Oat bran
- Brown rice
- Red lentils

- Split mung beans
- Kombu seaweed
- Apples
- Carrots
- Beets
- Leafy dark greens: a fresh assortment (lettuce, parsley, arugula, kale, dandelion, etc.)

- Lemons
- Cucumbers
- Tomatoes
- Raw sauerkraut
- Powdered spirulina (blue-green algae)
- An assortment of herbal noncaffeinated teas
- Laxative tea

Supplements—try to get all organic and vegan (no gelatin capsules):

- Aloe vera juice (preferably with pulp)
- Digestive enzymes
- Acidophilus (nondairy) in tablets or capsules

- Silica (horsetail) (helps promote strong and shiny hair and glowing skin)
- Multivitamins
- Vitamin B12

The following appliances will make your meal preparation easier:

- Blender or food processor
- Large soup pot (stainless steel—not aluminum or Teflon coated)
- Small saucepan (stainless steel—not aluminum or Teflon coated)

THE DIET PLAN

Breakfast

Upon rising:
- Take digestive enzymes and acidophilus on an empty stomach and drink 1–2 oz. of aloe vera juice.
- Drink a cup of herbal tea without any milk or sweeteners—chamomile, peppermint, and licorice are good options.

After 20 minutes:
- Eat a bowl of plain oatmeal without adding salt, sugar, soymilk, or any other kind of milk. After eating the oatmeal, take the multivitamin, B12, and silica tablets.

Lunch Snack
- If you feel hungry during the day, drink more herbal tea or some fresh vegetable or fruit juice (not bottled, canned, or processed) and lots of water.

Dinner
- 20 minutes before eating, drink an 8 oz. glass of room-temperature water, take digestive enzymes and acidophilus, and drink 1–2 oz. of aloe vera juice.
- Eat a bowl of kitchari.
- Eat a bowl of blended raw salad.
- Eat at least 2 tablespoons of raw sauerkraut.

How to make oatmeal:

Place ½ cup raw oats in a saucepan and add 2 cups of cold water. Bring to a boil, reduce heat to low, simmer for 10 minutes and serve. This makes a very creamy, souplike porridge.

How to make kitchari:

Measure out 1½ cups dry red lentils (or split mung beans) and ½ cup brown rice. Place in large soup pot and add 10 cups of water and a 4-inch piece of dry kombu seaweed. Bring to a boil and then simmer for about 1 hour. If you make a big batch, you can refrigerate it and use it over a few days. Just reheat and add more water if necessary.

How to make blended salad:

Place all the ingredients you might normally put in a large salad in a blender or food processor. Add 1 tablespoon lemon juice and 1 cup of cold water and blend. (Do not add any oil, vinegar, salt, or pepper!)

Here are some suggested ingredients for your blended salad:

- ½ apple
- ½ carrot
- ½ beet
- ½ cucumber
- 3 cherry tomatoes
- 6 romaine lettuce leaves
- 6 arugula leaves
- 1 teaspoon spirulina (blue-green algae) powder

Make your own sauerkraut:

It's actually easy. Check out the website Wild Fermentation (www.wildfermentation.com) for a recipe or buy some, but make sure it's raw.

Every night for the first week, drink a cup of herbal laxative tea before bedtime to get the elimination process going, then taper off and drink it only if you are having trouble eliminating in the morning.

CHAPTER 11

DELIGHTFUL DINING

Vegan Recipes for Human and
Animal People Alike

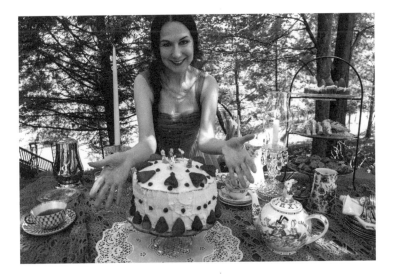

COOKING CAN BE A MAGICAL ACT, A POTENT ALCHEMICAL
process in which form transforms into another form.
The type of food you choose to prepare can provide
nourishment for your body and mind, as well as contribute to the health of others and the planet. Traditionally,
a yogi offered every activity, including cooking a meal,

to God before eating it. In the Bhagavad Gita, Krishna advises, "If you want to dispel ignorance and anxiety in your life, offer with love all of your actions to God, even the food you eat and the water you drink." Food and drink that has been offered to God is known in Sanskrit as *prasada*, which means "God's blessed gift."

patraṁ puṣpaṁ phalaṁ toyaṁ
yo me bhaktyā prayacchati
tad ahaṁ bhakty-upahṛtam
aśnāmi prayatātmanaḥ
BG 9.26

Whatever is offered to me with a pure loving heart, no matter if it is a leaf, a flower, a fruit, or a sip of water, I will accept it. The one who remembers me in this way is dear to me.

The following recipes come from my own kitchen. In this chapter, I have chosen to share with you some of the most favorite menu items I have created and served to the many human, cat, and birds guests who have come to dine with me in my home and at the Jivamuktea Café in New York City.

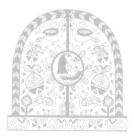

CHOCOLATE LAYER CAKE

INGREDIENTS:

- 3 cups all-purpose flour, plus more for dusting the pans
- 1½ cup sugar
- ½ cup unsweetened cocoa powder
- 1 teaspoon salt
- 2 teaspoons baking soda
- ⅔ cup safflower or canola oil
- 3 teaspoons vanilla extract
- 2 teaspoons white vinegar
- 2 cups ice-cold water
- Vanilla Sugar Icing (recipe follows)

PROCEDURE:

Step 1: Preheat oven to 350 degrees Fahrenheit.

Step 2: Grease the bottoms and sides of two 9-inch round cake pans with vegan margarine, then dust with flour.

Step 3: In a large bowl, place the flour, sugar, cocoa powder, salt, and baking soda and mix well with a whisk.

Step 4: Place the safflower or canola oil, vanilla extract, vinegar, and ice-cold water in a separate large bowl and mix well.

Step 5: Make a deep well in the center of the dry ingredients and pour in the wet ingredients. Stir with a large spoon just until all ingredients are mixed—do not overmix.

Step 6: Pour the batter into the prepared cake pans and bake for about 30 minutes or until a knife inserted in the center comes out clean. Remove from oven and set on a wire rack to cool.

Step 7: When the cake is completely cool, frost the cake with Vanilla Sugar Icing (see recipe below).

VANILLA SUGAR ICING

INGREDIENTS:
- 1 cup (2 sticks) vegan margarine, room temperature
- 4 cups confectioners' sugar
- 2 teaspoons vanilla extract
- 3 teaspoons vanilla soymilk (or almond milk)

PROCEDURE:

Step 1: In a large bowl, cream the margarine using a hand mixer. Add the confectioners' sugar, vanilla extract, and soymilk and mix with hand mixer on medium speed until thoroughly combined. The icing should be stiff.

Step 2: Spread a generous layer of icing on the top of one of the cakes, then place the other cake on top of the first iced layer. Spread a thin layer of icing on top of the second layer and all around the sides. Don't worry about getting crumbs mixed up with the icing.

Step 3: Put the cake and the leftover icing in the refrigerator for about 10–15 minutes. This will allow the icing on the cake to harden to a thin glaze, enabling you to finish icing the cake without crumbs getting mixed in.

Step 4: Take the icing and the cake out of the refrigerator and finish icing the cake.

Source: "Chocolate Layer Cake" and "Vanilla Sugar Icing" from *Simple Recipes for Joy: More Than 200 Delicious Vegan Recipes* by Sharon Gannon, copyright 2014 by Sharon Gannon. Used by permission of Penguin Books, an imprint of Penguin Publishing Group, a division of Penguin Random House LLC. All rights reserved.

VEGAN "POACHED EGGS" ON TOAST

INGREDIENTS:
- 2 slices bread
- 1 to 2 tablespoons flaxseed oil
- 1 tablespoon vegan butter
- 2 slices firm tofu cut in ¼-inch thick pieces
- Salt and freshly ground black pepper

PROCEDURE:

Step 1: Toast bread in a toaster. Spread flaxseed oil lavishly on the toast, then butter the toast lightly.

Step 2: Place 1 slice of tofu on each slice of toast, drizzle a few drops of flaxseed oil over the tofu, and sprinkle with salt and pepper to taste.

Serves 1

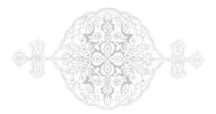

SPIRULINA MILLET

INGREDIENTS:

- 1 cup uncooked millet
- 2 cups water
- ¼ cup flaxseed oil
- ¼ cup powdered spirulina
- 1 tablespoon soy sauce, tamari, or Bragg Liquid Aminos

PROCEDURE:

Step 1: In a medium pot, place the millet in the water; cover and bring to a boil over high heat. Reduce the heat to low and simmer for about 20 minutes, until the liquid is absorbed. Turn off heat and let the cooked millet sit for about 10 minutes so it dries out some, then transfer it to a large bowl.

Step 2: Add the flaxseed oil and, using a large fork, mix well to coat the millet. Little by little, add the spirulina, using the fork to mix. Add the soy sauce, tamari, or Bragg Liquid Aminos, mixing well until the millet is bright green.

Serves 4–6

(NOTE: Many dogs and especially my cats are big fans of my Spirulina Millet recipe. They prefer it without the soy sauce and with a generous sprinkle of nutritional yeast flakes on top.)

LEAFY GREEN PESTO

INGREDIENTS:

- 4 cups densely packed fresh leafy greens (or use basil, parsley, arugula, spinach, cilantro, dandelion greens, wild mustard, or any combination of these)
- ⅓ cup raw sunflower seeds
- ⅓ cup olive oil
- 2 tablespoons mellow white miso
- 2 tablespoons lemon juice
- 2 tablespoons nutritional yeast
- ½ teaspoon black pepper

PROCEDURE:

Place all ingredients in a food processor and blend. For a chunkier pesto, be careful not to overblend.

Serves 4–6

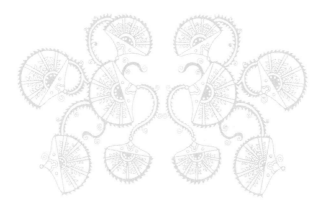

DAL

INGREDIENTS:

- 2 cups dried yellow, split mung beans (or red lentils)
- 8 cups water
- 2 tablespoons coconut oil
- 2-inch piece of fresh ginger, peeled and finely chopped
- 1 tablespoon cumin seeds*
- 1 tablespoon curry powder*
- 1 tablespoon turmeric powder*
- 1 teaspoon asafetida*
- 10 oz. can coconut milk
- 2 teaspoons salt
- ½ teaspoon dried crushed red pepper
- ¼ cup fresh or dried curry leaves*
- 1 cup fresh cilantro, chopped

PROCEDURE:

Step 1: Rinse the mung beans with cold water and drain well.

Step 2: Put mung beans in a large pot and add the water. Bring to a boil over high heat, then reduce to medium-low and cook for 1 hour.

Step 3: While mung beans are cooking, melt the coconut oil in a small frying pan over medium heat; add ginger and sauté about 1 minute, stirring often. Add cumin seeds, cover, and cook until you hear the seeds popping, then stir in curry powder, turmeric powder, and asafetida. Cook 1 more minute, set aside.

Step 4: When the mung beans are fully cooked and soft, transfer them to a food processor, stir in coconut milk, salt, and red pepper, and blend until smooth and creamy.

Step 5: Pour the blended mixture back into the large pot, add the cooked spices and curry leaves, and stir well. Continue cooking for another 5 minutes.

Step 6: Serve in bowls garnished with 1 tablespoon of chopped cilantro.

Serves 8–10

(NOTE: Ingredients marked with an asterisk may be found in an Indian grocery or ordered online if not available in your local market.)

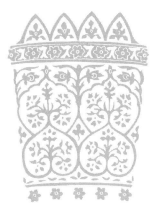

CURRY MISO VEGETABLE NOODLE SOUP

INGREDIENTS:

- 4 quarts (16 cups) water
- ¾ cup mellow white miso
- ½ cup tahini
- 1 bouillon cube (or 1 teaspoon powdered vegetable broth)
- 1 tablespoon toasted sesame oil
- 2 tablespoons tamari soy sauce
- 2 tablespoons curry powder
- 1 tablespoon turmeric powder
- 1 tablespoon cumin powder
- 2-inch piece of fresh ginger
- 2-inch square piece of dried kombu seaweed
- 2–3 large carrots, peeled and sliced
- 1 medium-size sweet potato or butternut squash, peeled and cubed
- 2 cups chopped white cabbage (sometimes called green cabbage), thinly sliced
- 15 oz. can garbanzo beans
- 10 oz. firm tofu, cut into small cubes
- 2 cups green beans, cut into 1-inch long pieces (or use frozen)
- 4 oz. dried bean thread noodles (also called glass or cellophane noodles)
- 1 cup fresh cilantro, finely chopped
- Hot-and-spicy toasted sesame oil

PROCEDURE:

Step 1: Fill a large pot with the water; heat to boil.

Step 2: In a medium-size bowl, place miso, tahini, bouillon, sesame oil, soy sauce, curry, turmeric, and cumin, add 1 cup of boiling water, and mix well until all ingredients are dissolved and blended. Best to use a small immersion mixer if you have one, or use a fork. Set aside.

Step 3: Peel ginger and chop into small pieces (about 2 tablespoons worth). Break the seaweed or cut with kitchen scissors into small pieces and add to pot of water.

Step 4: Peel carrots and cut into rounds, then slice each round in half (enough to fill 2 cups). Peel sweet potato (or butternut squash), cut into small cubes (enough to fill 2 cups). Thinly slice a wedge of white cabbage and then cut into smaller pieces (enough to fill 2 cups). Place all vegetables in the pot of water. Bring to a boil for about 10 minutes, then reduce heat to medium. Cook vegetables until soft (about 10–15 minutes).

Step 5: Add canned garbanzo beans (with liquid), cubed tofu, and green beans, and bring back to a boil (about 2–3 minutes).

Step 6: Add the miso-tahini mix to the pot, stir well, heat to just under boiling, and cook for 5 minutes, then add noodles and cook for another 1–2 minutes.

Step 7: Serve soup into individual bowls, garnish with generous helping of cilantro, and give guests the option to add a few drops of hot-and-spicy sesame oil to taste.

Serves 8–12

(NOTE: It might be helpful to use a pasta claw to serve the soup because the bean thread noodles are slippery.)

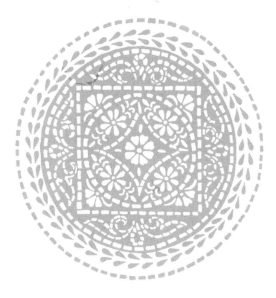

LASAGNA

INGREDIENTS:

- 2 ½ quarts (10 cups) water
- 2 teaspoons salt
- 2 oz. package dried lasagna noodles (at least 20 dry noodles)
- 1 tablespoon olive oil
- Two 25 oz. jars organic vegan marinara sauce (or use homemade)
- 14 oz. package firm tofu
- 1 tablespoon dried basil
- 1 tablespoon dried oregano
- 1 tablespoon dried rosemary
- 1 tablespoon dried thyme
- 2 cups firmly packed shredded fresh zucchini (or 4 cups firmly packed chopped fresh spinach leaves)
- 1 sweet red or yellow pepper, chopped into small pieces
- Two 8 oz. packages Daiya-brand vegan mozzarella-style shreds
- 1 cup nutritional yeast flakes
- ½ teaspoon crushed red pepper

PROCEDURE:

Step 1: Preheat oven to 375 degrees Fahrenheit.

Step 2: Place water in a large pan, add salt, and bring to a boil.

Step 3: Meanwhile, clear a space on your kitchen countertop and spread out a clean dish towel to receive the wet noodles.

Step 4: When water boils, add the lasagna noodles, following the directions on the noodle package (or boil noodles for 5 minutes, 5 noodles at a time). Use a timer and do not overcook. Remove each noodle from water with a flat slotted spoon and place on dish towel to dry. Immediately boil another batch of noodles.

Step 5: Use a 4-quart, 10- x 14- x 3-inch baking dish (or approximate size). Spread a small amount of olive oil on bottom of pan, then spread 4 tablespoons of prepared marinara sauce over it.

Step 6: In a medium-size bowl, place the block of tofu; using a large fork, break it up into crumbles. Mix in basil, oregano, rosemary, and thyme; set aside.

Step 7:

First layer: Carefully arrange a layer of lasagna noodles on the bottom of baking pan. It is okay for the noodles to overlap a bit to fit in the pan. Spread marinara sauce over the noodles. Place tofu-herb mixture on top of the sauce and cover with mozzarella-style cheese, then sprinkle about ¼ cup of nutritional yeast flakes on top of cheese.

Second layer: Carefully arrange another layer of noodles, spread marinara sauce over noodles, add shredded zucchini (or chopped spinach), then mozzarella cheese and ¼ cup of nutritional yeast flakes on top.

Third layer: Carefully arrange another layer of noodles, spread marinara sauce over noodles, and add chopped red pepper. Sprinkle crushed red pepper on top, then mozzarella cheese and ¼ cup of nutritional yeast flakes.

<u>Top layer</u>: Pour what remains of the marinara sauce and spread well over noodles, add mozzarella cheese and what remains of the nutritional yeast flakes.

Step 8: Cover with aluminum foil or heat-resistant lid. Bake 45 minutes covered, remove lid, and bake another 10 minutes uncovered, then let rest 10 minutes before serving.

Serves 8–10

(NOTE: Avoid using an aluminum pan; Pyrex glass or ceramic is nontoxic and best for distributing heat evenly. If your baking dish is smaller than the size suggested, simply reduce your layers to three, combining the second layer of zucchini or spinach with chopped red pepper.)

PAD THAI

INGREDIENTS:

- ½ lb. dried Pad Thai rice noodles (banh pho)
- 2-inch piece fresh ginger, peeled and chopped (2 tablespoons)
- 2 cups (about 2–3 carrots) julienned (cut into thin, 2-inch-long matchstick-size pieces)
- 1 cup thinly sliced white cabbage (or green cabbage)
- 4 oz. smoked tofu, cubed or cut into thin strips (use a commercial-brand product from SoyBoy, Taifun, or Soyganic, or make your own smoked tofu)
- 1 cup mung bean sprouts
- 1 cup cilantro, leaves and stems chopped into small pieces
- 1 cup romaine lettuce, finely chopped
- ¼ cup soy sauce
- 2 tablespoons tamarind chutney (or 2 tablespoons tamarind paste and 1 teaspoon sugar)
- 1 tablespoon Sriracha (or chili sauce)
- 3–4 tablespoons toasted sesame oil (or any vegetable oil)
- Nutritional yeast to taste
- ¼ cup ground roasted peanuts
- Fresh lemon or lime wedges (at least ¼ per serving)

PROCEDURE:

Step 1: Put noodles in a large bowl and cover with hot water. Let soak until just pliable but not mushy, about 6–8 minutes. Drain the noodles in a colander, rinse with cold water, shake off any excess water, and let sit until ready to add to stir-fry vegetables.

Step 2: Meanwhile, prepare ginger, carrots, cabbage, tofu, bean sprouts, cilantro, and lettuce. Set aside.

Step 3: In a small bowl, whisk the soy sauce with tamarind chutney and Sriracha.

Step 4: In a large wok or skillet, heat sesame oil until simmering. Add ginger and cook 1 minute, then add carrots and cabbage and cook over high heat, stirring occasionally, for about 5 minutes. Add tofu and continue to cook for about 2 minutes. Stir in noodles and cook until heated through, about 1 minute. Add sauce and mix until noodles and vegetables are evenly coated and the sauce has thickened slightly, about 2–3 minutes.

Step 5: Turn off heat. Mix in cilantro and bean sprouts.

Step 6: Prepare plates by first putting about ¼ cup finely chopped lettuce on each plate. Use a pasta claw to serve the Pad Thai noodles, placing a helping over the chopped lettuce. Top with a generous sprinkle of nutritional yeast and peanuts. Serve with fresh lemon or lime wedges.

Serves 4

And now something for the birds:

VEGAN WILD BIRD SUET

INGREDIENTS:
- 3½ cup wild birdseed
- 1 cup quick organic oats
- ½ cup organic corn meal
- 1½ cup organic coconut oil (refined-neutral taste)
- ¾ cup organic peanut butter

PROCEDURE:

Step 1: In a large bowl, mix dry ingredients together.

Step 2: In a small pan, melt coconut oil and peanut butter.

Step 3: Pour the oil and peanut butter over dry ingredients and mix together.

Step 4: Spoon into molds (plastic Tupperware containers work well). Flatten into a shape that will fit into your suet cage.

Step 5: Freeze to set (at least 5 hours).

Step 6: Place one "brick" in suet cage and hang outside for bird friends to enjoy.

(NOTE: Only make in cold winter months; otherwise, the oil will melt.)

Here are a few special menu items for cats (and dogs, too) you may want to try:

Contrary to popular belief, I have discovered that cats are omnivores and not strict carnivores; they enjoy eating vegetables. Even though I do not feed my cat companions a vegan diet, about 75 percent of what is in their dinner bowl is plant-based and always organic. I do not recommend a strict vegan diet for cats, but dogs, on the other hand, can thrive on a vegan diet. Cats are unable to synthetize the essential amino acid taurine from plant sources, while dogs, like human beings and other primates, can. If you're interested in exploring this subject more, see my book *Cats and Dogs Are People Too!*, which goes into detail about feline nutrition and a lot more.

STEAMED VEGGIES

INGREDIENTS:
- Cauliflower (or broccoli, green beans, zucchini, or asparagus)
- Nutritional yeast flakes

PROCEDURE:

Step 1: Choose any one of the vegetables listed above or make a medley of all five. Cut into cat-bite-size pieces and steam (about 3–5 minutes). Most cats like their veggies a bit crisp, so don't overcook.

Step 2: Remove from steamer and cool.

Step 3: Place veggies in cat serving bowl and sprinkle with a generous sprinkle of yeast flakes.

KASHA DELIGHT

INGREDIENTS:
- ¼ cup cooked kasha (buckwheat groats)
- ¼ cup frozen or canned green peas
- ¼ cup raw tempeh, cut into very small cat-bite-size pieces
- 1 tablespoon flaxseed oil
- ¼ cup alfalfa sprouts
- 1 tablespoon nutritional yeast flakes

PROCEDURE:

Step 1: Cook kasha according to package directions. Cook green peas until soft; if using canned peas, no need to cook them.

Step 2: In a medium-size mixing bowl, place cooked kasha, peas, raw tempeh, and flaxseed oil; mix together with a fork.

Step 3: Place mixture in cat serving bowl; top with alfalfa sprouts and a generous sprinkle of yeast flakes.

RAW ZUCCHINI-CARROT SALAD

INGREDIENTS:
- 1 tablespoon raw zucchini, shredded (measurement is approximate)
- 1 tablespoon raw carrot, peeled and shredded (measurement is approximate)
- ½ teaspoon flaxseed oil (or melted refined coconut oil); use neutral-taste variety
- ½ teaspoon nutritional yeast flakes
- ¼ teaspoon spirulina powder

PROCEDURE:

Step 1: Using a stainless-steel vegetable shredder, shred about 1 tablespoon of raw zucchini and raw carrot.

Step 2: Mix zucchini and carrot shreds with flaxseed oil.

Step 3: Place in bowl and sprinkle yeast flakes and spirulina on top.

Sharon Gannon is the most impassioned and truthful vegan chef and yogi alive today on Mother Earth.
—JOE SPONZO, PERSONAL CHEF TO STING AND TRUDIE STYLER

Sharon's recipes are from the heart, always keeping the well-being of others in mind—both human and animal. She is a tireless voice for the voiceless and a great cook, too!
—JENNY BROWN, CO-FOUNDER OF THE WOODSTOCK FARM ANIMAL SANCTUARY

CHAPTER 12

FREQUENTLY ASKED QUESTIONS

In THIS CHAPTER, I ANSWER QUESTIONS REGARDING YOGA and veganism. These inquiries all came from real-life interactions I have had with others, instigating me to delve deeper into my own mind and heart through the process of compassionate contemplation and critical thinking. The questions have provoked and inspired me to grow, transcending my own limitations and what I thought I knew, to arrive at answers that are sincere and helpful. Through reading both the questions and answers, your perceptions will hopefully be expanded, and you will feel encouraged to continue your own investigation into the connections between the subjects of yoga and veganism.

Through my experience, I have come to recognize that there are basically four reasons a person might choose to become vegan: for **health**, out of concern for the **environment**, for **animal rights**, and for **spiritual realization**. Even though many of us will see these reasons as overlapping, the Q&A falls under those four headings for easy reference.

— HEALTH —

I did not become a vegetarian for my health.
I did it for the health of the chickens.
—Isaac Bashevis Singer

It's not one set of dietary guidelines for improving your performance as an athlete, another one for reversing heart disease, a different one for reversing diabetes, a different one for reversing prostate cancer. It's the same for all of them—a plant-based diet.
—Dean Ornish, MD

1. *Q: How can I get enough protein if I eat a vegan diet?*
A: The required daily amount (RDA) of protein is 50–70 grams, which is easily met by eating a wide assortment of plant foods. It is a myth that only animal products contain protein. There is protein in beans and grains as well as in almonds, broccoli, mushrooms, avocados, and even potatoes. There is another myth that says you must carefully combine proteins from plant sources in each meal to meet the RDA. This is not true. Simply eat a variety of plant foods over the course of a day, and you will meet your protein requirements. Read the book *Hope's Edge*, by Frances Moore Lappé and Anna Lappé, for more information.

2. Q: Can I get vitamin B12 on a vegan diet?

A: A vegan must rely on getting adequate vitamin B12 from a supplement or from eating foods that have been fortified with vitamin B12. If we weren't so dirt-conscious, we would obtain adequate vitamin B12 from soil, air, water, and bacteria, but we meticulously wash and peel our vegetables now—and with good reason, as we can't be sure our soil is not contaminated with pesticides and herbicides. Today, "aged" foods like sauerkraut, miso, and tempeh are fermented in hygienically sanitized stainless-steel vats to ensure cleanliness, so we can no longer be sure they will provide us with the B12 we need. Vegans should not mess around with this issue. To guarantee that you are getting the tiny amount (2.5 micrograms) you need per day, take a supplement and/or drink fortified soymilk or rice milk. Read the book *Becoming Vegan*, by Brenda Davis, RD, and Vesanto Melina, MS, RD, for more information.

3. Q: Don't I need to drink milk to get enough calcium?

A: No. In fact, drinking milk and eating dairy products can rob your body of calcium and contribute to osteoporosis. If you eat dark-green leafy vegetables like kale, collards, and mustard greens, you can get enough calcium from a vegan diet. Beans, tofu, cabbage, and broccoli are additional sources of calcium. If you doubt that you are meeting the 1,000-milligram RDA, include calcium-fortified foods like fruit juice, cereals, or soy or grain beverages, or take a supplement. Also, the weight-bearing aspect of yoga asana practice contributes to bone density and health. Sunlight is essential to the body's ability to absorb calcium from the food you are eating. Make sure you receive adequate vitamin D every day through sunlight. About fifteen to twenty minutes of sun on the face and hands is usually enough for most of us. Read the book *CalciYum!*, by David and Rachelle Bronfman, for more information and recipes.

4. Q: Aren't we hardwired to eat meat?

A: No, eating meat is a learned behavior. It is like a software program downloaded into our computer-like brains. It is not part of the hard drive (or the heart drive). How can I say that with total certainty? Because if eating meat was hardwired in us, then a person like me, who is a vegan, would not be able to survive. And yet I do exist, and many others like me do also, all of us thriving on a totally meat-free, dairy-free, plant-based vegan diet. So, here we are—the living proof.

5. Q: Aren't humans biologically designed to be meat eaters or at least omnivores?

A: The anatomical and physiological facts suggest no. We have small, flat mouths with small teeth. We don't have long, sharp canines to tear flesh. We have incisors in the front to bite and molars along the sides to chew and grind fruits and vegetables. Our teeth aren't strong enough to chew and crush hard things like raw bones, whereas carnivores can. We have a rotating jaw that moves from side to side, another useful feature for grinding plants. Carnivores and omnivores have hinge-joint jaws that open and close. They don't normally chew their food well before swallowing, and they don't need to. Unlike us, they don't have an abundance of the enzyme *ptyalin* in their saliva, which breaks down complex carbohydrates found only in plant foods. Once we have chewed and swallowed our food, it travels through a very long digestive tract, although not as long as that of our herbivore friends—the cows, horses, and sheep. Meat-eating species, comparatively, have short intestinal tracts, which allow them to move food through their systems quickly so as not to allow rotting flesh to stagnate and cause disease.

Because we lack sharp claws, aren't very fast on our feet, and aren't exactly endowed with lightning reflexes, it would be very difficult if not impossible for us to run down an animal, catch it with our bare hands, and tear through its fur and skin in order to eat it. Biologically, we are designed to be frugivorous herbivores eating mainly fruits, seeds, roots, and leaves.

Humans do not need to eat the flesh of other animals to exist, whereas some animals are carnivores and cannot survive by eating only vegetables. Humans, on the other hand, eat meat only out of choice. We have been conditioned, taught, and coerced by the agents of our culture (parents, grandparents, advertisers, food critics, etc.) to eat the flesh and drink the milk of other animals. Because of this conditioning, which has occurred over a long period (thousands of years), we have developed addictive eating habits and blinded ourselves to the facts of our biological system and its true needs. As Neal Barnard says, "The beef industry has contributed to more American deaths than all the wars of this century, all natural disasters, and all automobile accidents combined. If beef is your idea of 'real food for real people,' you'd better live real close to a real good hospital."[66]

6. Q: Why have we been told that eating meat and drinking milk are good for us and make strong bones and teeth, etc., and now we are learning that it's just the opposite?

A: Most people are gullible and will believe anything that is presented to them with authority and confidence. Stage magicians, actors, politicians, journalists, and businesspeople all know the power of presentation. The wizards in the fields of advertising and publicity understand this rule and through persuasive language and seductive packaging can convince others of just about anything. Selling products is more about making money than making our lives healthier or happier.

7. Q: I just want to practice yoga for the physical benefits. Why should I be concerned with veganism, the environment, or political activism?

A: What could be more physical than what you eat, where you live, and with whom you live?

8. Q: How does the practice of yoga and veganism help integrate a person's body and mind?

A: By bringing about a more holistic perception of who you are and where you are in the bigger picture of the

---

66 Physicians Committee for Responsible Medicine, https://www.pcrm.org.

world. When you practice yoga for what it was originally intended—to bring about enlightenment—you come to see your physical body as an extension of and not separate from your mind, emotions, or soul. The practice results in a person becoming a holy being, a more whole, integrated, more confident, and most importantly a happier person—no longer perceiving their body as separate from the rest of their being, and even further more no longer seeing their body as separate from other bodies. You come to understand that what you do to another, you ultimately do to yourself. You come to see the power of your actions and that no one is insignificant to the whole scheme of things. The actions that each of us take matter to the whole world; in fact, it is our individual actions that create the world we live in.

9. Q: *What emotional and mental health benefits do we gain by living life rooted in compassion and spiritual activism?*
A: A sense of cynicism and hopelessness, so prevalent these days, destroys our enthusiasm, our passion for life. *Enthusiasm* comes from a Greek root word, *enthous*, which means "be possessed by God or divinely inspired." Through compassion and spiritual activism, enthusiasm is ignited in one's mind and heart resulting in peace of mind, a loving heart, clarity of purpose, joyfulness, optimism, and true Self-confidence—confidence that comes not from the desire for the recognition of your accomplishments but from being a part of something bigger, being a joyful instrument for love.

10. *Q: Are there vegan countries or vegan areas or vegan communities? What is the result in these places or groups that have taken up this diet? Are they proving any of these theories you are proposing?* *A:* To my knowledge, there are no countries where every citizen is a vegan. I have, however, visited a few vegan communities, among them the Tree of Life Center US in Patagonia, Arizona.67

My own home is a vegan community, as is the Jivamukti Yoga global community of teachers and students, which numbers a minimum of 20,000 people as of 2020, considered thriving on a healthy vegan diet. I am not a medical doctor, nor do I work for the EPA as a professional environmentalist; my main expertise is in the area of yoga. The "theories" I am proposing are kindness, compassion, love, and respect for others—all others including other animals.

With this book, I am investigating what is found in the classical yoga system of Patanjali and how those ideas might be applicable to us in our present time. In regard to health, Patanjali says that if you refrain from abusing others sexually, you will enjoy vitality and good health yourself (see chapter 6, "Brahmacharya: Good Sex"). It seems to me that this naturally points to a vegan diet, because we sexually abuse all animals that are raised as livestock to be eaten. The old term for this in our global culture is *animal husbandry*. So, the practice

---

67 Gabriel Cousens, "Success Stories," http://www.treeoflifecenterus.com/success-stories. Further examples: Vegan Flourish, "Vegan Communities," https://www.veganflourish. com/vegan-communities-directory; Vegan Runners, https://www.veganrunners. org.uk. See also *The Game Changers: Benefits of Optimizing Health*, https://www. gamechangersmovie.com/benefits/optimizing-health.

of raping, sexually abusing, and manipulating animals is an old farming practice that has been sanctioned for thousands of years all over the world. With the ideas expressed in the yogic scriptures (call them theories if you like), I am questioning those practices.

Can I prove that a vegan diet, a diet that does not involve rape and sexual abuse of animals, results in good health? All I can say, in all certainty, is that I am almost seventy years old and have been a vegan since my early thirties; I have no major health issues, am very physically fit, and have experienced no decline in energy level. Even so, I do not expect to live forever. No matter what diet you eat, it will not grant you immortality.

11. Q: What about Eskimos?

A: Everyone, without exception, must reap what they have sown. There is no escape from the law of karma. Because of the shortage of available vegetables, Arctic-dwelling Eskimos eat a large amount of meat and animal fat. They also have one of the highest incidences of heart disease and osteoporosis[68] in the world and, in general, short life spans.[69] That's something to consider.

---

68 R. Mazess, "Bone Mineral Content of North Alaskan Eskimos," *American Journal of Clinical Nutrition* 9 (1974): 916–925.

69 Geoff Bond. *Deadly Harvest: The Intimate Relationship Between Our Health and Our Food* (New York: Square One, 2007), 91.

— ENVIRONMENT —

When we poison the water, we poison ourselves.
—JOHN ROBBINS

By eating meat and dairy, we share the responsibility of climate change, the destruction of our forests, and the poisoning of our air and water. The simple act of becoming a vegan will make a difference in the health of our planet.
—THICH NHAT HANH

12. Q: Can someone be a meat-eating environmentalist?
A: If that someone is a human being, in my opinion, no; it is a contradiction in terms. To be an environmentalist is to care about the environment and care about life on planet Earth. The raising of animals for food and all that it entails is the single most destructive force impacting our planet's fragile ecosystems. Our planet simply cannot sustain the greed of billions of human beings who are eating other animals.

13. Q: If we all become vegans, will there be enough vegetables to feed all of us?
A: If we stop feeding grain to livestock, we will have enough food to feed all the starving human beings in the world. A reduction of meat consumption by only 10 percent would yield enough grain to feed all the humans who starve to death each year worldwide—about sixty

million.[70] Buddhist teacher Thich Nhat Hanh says, "Every day, 40,000 children die in the world for lack of food. We who overeat in the West, who are feeding grains to animals to make meat, are eating the flesh of these children."[71]

14. Q: If yoga teaches us that all of life is sacred, what is the difference if I eat a carrot or a hamburger?

A: Yes, all of life is sacred, and there is scientific evidence supporting the idea that plants have feelings. However, in the Yoga Sutras, Patanjali gives ahimsa, or nonharming, as a "practice," which implies that it can never be perfected. You practice doing your best to cause the least amount of harm. He also recommends aparigraha, the practice of not being greedy, or taking too much. The animals we eat consume large quantities of vegetables, so when you eat those animals, you are consuming not only the animals but also all the vegetables that those animals have been eating.

Additionally, animals raised for human consumption require a lot of food and land. It takes eight or nine cows a year to feed one average meat eater. Each cow eats one acre of green plants, soybeans, and corn.[72] Most of the plants grown to be fed to farm animals are heavily saturated with pesticides and herbicides and have been genetically modified, all of which contributes

70 Boyce Resenberger. "Curb on US Waste Urged to Help World's Hungry," *New York Times* (Oct. 25 1974).
71 Thich Nhat Hanh. *Creating True Peace: Ending Violence in Yourself, Your Family, Your Community, and the World* (New York: Simon & Schuster, 2003) 77.
72 Marc Bekoff, *Strolling with Our Kin: Speaking for and Respecting Voiceless Animals* (New York: Lantern, 2000), 70.

to the pollution and death of our environment. In terms of causing the least amount of harm, a vegan diet is superior because a vegan eats the plants directly instead of eating the animals who were fed plants.

15. *Q: Isn't the real problem human overpopulation rather than meat eating?*

A: Human population growth is a problem in that most humans consume more than they need. The Earth's resources are now strained to sustain the needs and wants of the human population, which continues to escalate. The wealthier countries have curbed their population growth, in some cases to zero, while people in poorer or so-called developing countries give birth to many more babies on average. In the United States, the average is two children per family, while in Africa it is five.[73] On the surface, the statistic seems to indicate that Africans are having way too many kids and are taxing the Earth's resources, while American kids are born into families that are able to take care of them. However, the average American child consumes roughly the same resources as fifteen African children.[74] So, when an American family says they only have two children, they are actually consuming the resources of an African family of thirty children! Furthermore, those American children

---

73 Erin Duffin, "Average Number of Own Children Under 18 in Families with Children in the United States from 1960 to 2018," Statista, https://www.statista.com/statistics/718084/average-number-of-own-children-per-family; The Conversation. "Why African Families Are Larger Than Those of Other Continents (October 11, 2017), https://www.theconversation.com/why-african-families-are-larger-than-those-of-other-continents-84611.

74 Roger-Mark Desouza, John S. Williams, and Frederick Meyerson, "Critical Links: Population, Health and the Environment," *Population Bulletin* 58.3 (2003), https://www.prb.org/criticallinkspopulationhealthandtheenvironmentpdf340kb.

will be indoctrinated into a lifestyle that teaches them to consume more than they need. Human overconsumption is a greater problem than human population growth, and meat eating is a big part of that problem. Some well-to-do parents may say, "I have a right to have as many children as I want because I can take care of them." That may be so, but can the Earth take care of them?

16. Q: How can being a vegan environmentalist contribute to living in harmony with the Earth?

A: When your actions are motivated by a desire to enhance the lives of others and even to enhance the Earth Herself, then you begin to glimpse your true cosmic potential as a member of the universe. You consider your actions before you take them. You tune in and try to see the potential outcome of your choices and you try to be a player in the ensemble—a positive contributor to the happiness of the planet and all her creatures. You are a kind and benevolent presence in the lives of others and see yourself as part of the family of life. You actively free yourself of the debilitating notion of being a superior being that sees others as existing to be exploited by you. Thinking that the Earth belongs to you because you are a human being does not contribute to a harmonious relationship for you with the Earth or with others. Instead, it causes you to feel disconnected. The cultivation of humility heals the disease of disconnection, which is an epidemic in the world today. *Humility* comes from the Latin root *humilitas*, meaning "humble, from the Earth, low to the ground, unpretentious." From this humble root, the word *human* comes. So, to be human means to be humble. Wow! That's something for all us human beings to remember and reflect on.

17. Q: In a recent study on global population growth, scientists were said to be scrambling to devise a diet plan that could feed 10 billion people by 2050. Is the planet really able to sustain 10 billion people, even if they all consume a vegan diet? Shouldn't we just make more of all kinds of food to meet this demand?

A: A new report, published in the British medical journal the *Lancet*,[75] claims to do just that. The report was compiled by a group of thirty scientists from around the world who study nutrition or food policy. For three years, they deliberated with the intent of creating recommendations that governments could adopt to meet the challenge of feeding a growing world population. In conclusion, their report recommends a largely plant-based diet, with small, occasional allowances for meat, dairy, and sugar.

But I'm not sure what they mean by "small, occasional allowances." From observation, it seems that our species has lost its ability to self-regulate; most people don't know when enough is enough and would not be able to determine on their own what a "small" amount of meat or dairy products actually means. We are not good at restricting ourselves when it comes to consumption. Any attempt to restrict our ability to eat, buy, or

---

75 Walter Willet et al. "Food in the Anthropocene: The EAT-Lancet Commission on Healthy Diets from Sustainable Food Systems," *The Lancet Commissions* 393:10170, Jan. 16, 2019, https://doi.org/10.1016/S0140-6736(18)31788-4.

procreate has been met with opposition and falls into a human rights debate. Perhaps we should rethink our ideas about human rights. At present, "human rights" seems to mean "the freedom to do as you like, as long as you have the money and power to do it—without any responsibility to others or the planet."

18. Q: It seems really strange that the government would subsidize big industries like meat and dairy if they are bad for our health and environment. Are they really that bad, and should the government perhaps subsidize what you consider environmentally friendly, good industries?
A: Yes they are "that" bad. But it comes down to money. If something is cheap, people tend to buy more of it, but with every purchase of cheap meat and dairy products there are hidden costs: costs to our health, costs to the environment, and, of course, costs to the animals—costing them their freedom, happiness, and lives. Meat, dairy, eggs, and fish are big business, contributing billions to the global economy. These industries hire powerful lobbyists to influence government policies. Politicians are generally not known for their dietary acumen, and they often peddle their political favors for election contributions. The U.S. government spends $38 billion each year to subsidize the meat and dairy industries but only $17 million to subsidize fruits and vegetables annually.[76]

---

76 David Robinson Simon. "10 Things We Wish Everyone Knew About the Meat Industry," PETA (Dec. 6, 2013), https://www.peta.org/living/food/10-things-wish-everyone-knew-meat-dairy-industries.

It is a travesty that our economy is based on something that is destroying ourselves and our planet. It would be to our ultimate advantage if, instead, we could support producers of plant-based foods. What can we do immediately? Vote with our pocketbooks. Make the choice to buy less or, better yet, no meat, fish, dairy, and eggs, and replace those things with healthy plant foods. Get educated and share what you know with your family and friends. For more information and solutions, get the book *Meatonomics*, by David Robinson Simon and visit Meatonomics: The Bizarre Economics of Meat and Dairy (www.meatonomics.com/the-book), the website the meat industry doesn't want you to see.

19. *Q: Shouldn't we, as spiritual practitioners, try to live a more simple life and just eat normal food and not be picky? Veganism seems so complicated!*
A: It is a testament to the effectiveness of advertising campaigns funded by the animal-user industries that a diet that is bad for us and harmful to the planet is thought of as "normal" and a diet that promotes health, happiness, and well-being is thought of as alternative, abnormal, or faddish. In fact, these days it is relatively easy to find vegan options in many restaurants and supermarkets, though you may have to ask. Moreover, the fact is that it is much more complicated to confine, raise, feed, slaughter, process, package, and market an animal for food than it is to grow plants.

20. *Q: At least if we choose to eat fish, it's cleaner for the environment and we aren't contributing to* *the ecological toll that eating beef or pork is causing, right?*

A: Wrong. Fishing is taking a huge toll on the planet's ecosystem. We are emptying the oceans, seas, lakes, and rivers as we fish them dry. Large factory trawlers indiscriminately scrape and haul up everything from the ocean floor, along with everyone unfortunate enough to get caught in the nets. Roughly one-third of what is dragged in is not profitable fish, but other sea animals, including turtles, whales, dolphins, seals, and sea birds[77]—beings referred to by the fishing industry as by-catch. Severely traumatized and wounded, these animals are subsequently thrown back into the ocean, dead or dying.

To meet the huge consumer demand for fish, the industry can no longer rely on hunting wild fish. Now we are doing to fish what was done to wild cows, sheep, goats, chickens, and ducks thousands of years ago: We are confining them in holding pens. These floating fish farms or hatcheries, like their land equivalents, are sites for genetic engineering. They contribute to polluting the ocean with toxic excrement and residue, as any other farm would. Many genetically "altered" fish escape from the confines of the crowded floating concentration camps to mingle and mate with their wild fish cousins, causing horrible and irreversible damage to wild species.

Today's fishing industry supplies land farms with fish as well. Over 50 percent of the fish caught are fed to livestock on factory farms and "regular" farms[78] as an ingredient in the enriched "feed meal" fed to livestock.

---

77 Tuttle, *The World Peace Diet*, 102.
78 S. J. Holt. "The Food Resources of the Ocean," *Scientific American* 221 (1969): 178–194.

Farm animals, like cows, who by nature are vegans, are routinely force-fed fish as well as the flesh, blood, and manure of other animals. It may take 16 pounds of grain to make 1 pound of beef, but it also takes 100 pounds of fish to make that 1 pound of beef.[79]

21. Q: I grew up on a dairy farm, and I know that cow manure, for example, is very healthy for the soil and for growing good crops. It seems like dairy farming is part of a natural cycle that is good for the soil and the environment. And using cow manure reduces the use of pesticides. What's wrong with this?

A: From an environmental perspective, there is a lot wrong with it. An average cow produces 100 pounds a day of manure. There are about 10 million dairy cows in the United States and 250 million cows producing milk globally.[80] That is a lot of manure being produced daily, and what happens to it? Manure releases methane gas, contributing to global warming. Most dairy cows are not fed healthy diets, so their poop is heavily contaminated and poses serious environmental problems to our water, soil, and air. Dangerous pathogens like salmonella, listeria and *E. coli*, as well as parasites, can be found in manure. Most dairy cows are fed antibiotics, hormones, and other drugs; these pharmaceuticals pass into their manure, eventually contaminating the soil and water.

Furthermore, in order to get a cow to produce enough milk to make her profitable, she is fed hormones

79 Watson, "Consider the Fishes," *VegNews*, 27.
80 U.S. Department of Agriculture (USDA) Natural Resources Conservation Service, "Animal Manure Management," USDA (December 1995), http://www.nrcs.usda.gov/wps/portal/nrcs/detail/null/?cid=nrcs143_014211.

and enriched food that contains animal products, especially fish. Our oceans are in decline, and for many reasons, farmed fish is not the answer; one is that it takes more than 5 pounds of wild fish to produce 1 pound of farmed fish, and many farmed fish are also fed GMO corn and soy.[81] Farmed fish are not healthy fish. They are overcrowded and fed lots of antibiotics. These antibiotics are passed into the bodies of the dairy cows or whoever ends up eating the fish that is passed out in their manure.

These are just a few environmental hazards connected with dairy farming and the inevitable poop excreted by the cows. But perhaps the more serious ethical question is "Should we be sanctioning the enslavement, sexual abuse, and murder of mothers?" A cow, like a human woman, is the female of her species. Bulls and steers are males and do not have breasts, produce milk, or have babies. A cow produces milk when she is pregnant and has just given birth to a baby. A dairy farm, whether it is a small farm or a large industrial complex, is a cruel place that produces immeasurable suffering as well as mountains of con-taminated manure and lagoons of toxic urine.

22. *Q: I heard that NASA has recently warned that water shortage, not meat eating, is likely to be the key environmental challenge of this century. So, really, isn't polluting our water the real problem?*

---

81 Cowspiracy, "The Facts," https://www.cowspiracy.com/facts.

A: Access to fresh water is a growing concern—all the more reason to be vegan. The meat and dairy industries consume more water than any other industry, and raising animals for food is the biggest polluter of water. It takes more than 2,400 gallons of water to produce 1 pound of beef, while producing 1 pound of tofu requires only 244 gallons of water.[82] (Tofu is just one example to show that growing vegetables takes less water than raising animals.)

23. *Q: Does pushing for a vegan world mean that hunting is excluded? How do you control animal overpopulation? Or what about an environment where not enough plants can be grown due to cold or hot weather, and you need to hunt for your food?*

A: In human society, murder is not considered a valid solution for old age. Wild animals are not immortal; like all of us, they do die. And like us, I would suspect, they would prefer to die of natural causes rather than to be violently murdered. I do think there is an overpopulation problem—too many human beings—but murder is not the answer. There is actually not an overpopulation of wild animals. Wild animals are becoming more and more scarce and dying of starvation, and many are becoming extinct. Yes, there are many reports of deer, elk, raccoons, and Canada geese walking down the main streets of many towns, and deer are grazing on suburban lawns and raccoons are rummaging through our garbage cans, and this may lead people to think

---

82 PETA, "Meat and the Environment," https://www.peta.org/issues/animals-used-for-food/meat-environment.

that the wild-animal population is out of control, but what actually is happening is that we are cutting down forests and paving over fields and meadows to make roads, shopping malls, and houses in places that once provided homes and food for wild animals. We have displaced them, made them homeless and hungry. They have nowhere to go because we are everywhere.

To address your question about needing to hunt for your food, perhaps a better solution than murdering defenseless animals who are just trying to eke out a living finding enough food to survive in habitats that have been compromised by human encroachment would be to learn to hunt for nourishing food in the supermarket. These days, it is the rare human being who needs to hunt for his or her food by hunting others.

24. Q: How does the United States compare to other countries in the world on veganism? Are we at least making progress?

A: I am seeing progress all over the world: Families are becoming vegan, people are making home-cooked organic food for their dogs, and new vegan restaurants are opening every day in some country in the world. Airplanes are offering vegan meals, and there are vegan-cooking classes in Cambodia. Yogis are feeding free vegan lunches to schoolchildren in India. Fashion designers are dropping fur, wool, and leather from their product lines and opting to use only vegan materials, and animal sanctuaries all over the world are rescuing and caring for pigs, chickens, cows, donkeys, dogs, and more. Ultimately, the question is not "What are others doing or not doing?" It is always "What am I doing?" If we want to know how the world is doing, just look at what's on our own plates.

25. Q: A lot of people think it would be expensive to make the kind of changes you're suggesting. If the richer, first-world countries move more quickly toward a more vegan diet, would we pressure poorer third-world countries to do so?
A: It is more expensive not to make the change to veganism. For many years now, affluent countries have been exporting their meat and dairy eating habits without compunction to poorer countries whose traditional diets were mainly plant based.

— ANIMAL RIGHTS —

The day will come when men such as I look on the murder of animals the way they now look on the murder of men.
—Leonardo da Vinci

We know we cannot be kind to animals until we stop exploiting them—exploiting animals in the name of science, exploiting animals in the name of sport, exploiting animals in the name of fashion, and, yes, exploiting animals in the name of food.
—César Chávez

26. Q: What would farm animals do if we stop eating them and let them go free? Where will they go?

They've been domesticated for thousands of years; they don't know how to live on their own. Wouldn't it be a form of cruelty not to take care of them?

A: This is the same argument that white American slave owners gave in the 1800s when they tried to defend their right to own slaves. Yes, we have robbed these animals of their wildness, and they might not be able to revert to a feral state if all the doors of all the factory farms were opened. We have severely altered these animals biologically and emotionally, depriving them of any opportunity to develop skills with which to live with one another and their environment. This process of degradation has been going on for thousands of generations. The first step is to stop abusing these beings—stop breeding them through cruel, artificial means. It may be unrealistic to let them all go free right now, but it is realistic to acknowledge that as a species, we human beings are quite ingenious. If we give serious consideration to this problem, we will no doubt find solutions and eventually free these animals. When we do, we will free ourselves.

27. *Q: No one was so up in arms about meat eating until recently, with the rise of industrialized farming and the cruel practices common in today's factory farms. Couldn't we go back to a simpler way of raising animals for food and support only small family-owned farms where animals are treated humanely?*

A: Farms, whether small or large, are places where slaves are kept. The animals are fattened up to be eaten, or exploited for their ability to make honey or milk, or for their fur, wool, or body parts; they are kept as breeders to produce more animals who can in turn be exploited and ultimately sold, slaughtered, and eaten. Some people may argue that if the animals are treated humanely prior to being slaughtered, this justifies their confinement and slaughter. Is it ethical to rob beings of their freedom but give them a comfortable prison and provide them with food until they become fat enough to be slaughtered? Any way you look at it, farms are places where animals are kept in preparation to be slaughtered and ultimately eaten as food. The question might be put this way: Is it really that much better to make friends with animals before you kill them than to treat them as nameless, faceless objects before you kill them? From a yogic point of view, one must weigh the karmic consequences of perceiving others as mere objects to be used and the consequences of profiting from the suffering of others.

28. Q: Is there a difference between animal rights and animal welfare?

A: Yes. Animal rights activists believe that animals exist for their own reasons, not to be used by human beings. Some animal rights activists take an abolitionist stance and feel that we have no moral right to exploit animals for any reason. Activist Ingrid Newkirk sums it up like this: "Animals are not ours to eat, wear, experiment on, or use for entertainment or for any exploitative purpose." Animal welfarists, on the other hand, do not believe that the lives of animals are important for their own sake. They believe that if we take care of animals and see to their welfare by providing them with a quality of life that gives them the appearance of happiness and health, it is okay to exploit them for our own purposes. Welfarists are concerned with the quality of the animals' lives before or even during their slaughter and want animals to be treated, and slaughtered, "humanely." Welfarists don't necessarily feel that it is wrong for humans to use animals for our own purposes.

29. Q: Are animals a lower life-form than humans?
A: It has been an obsession of human beings to create a hierarchy that places the human species on top and lumps all the other animals together beneath us. The resulting speciesism allows us to look on animals as less deserving of all manner of rights and considerations than humans. To support this lower status, humans have argued that animals act instinctively, don't have souls, don't feel physical pain like we do, and lack self-consciousness, cognitive intelligence, emotional feelings, morality, and ethics. In fact, numerous scientific laboratory tests and field observations have led to the conclusion that animals are conscious, intelligent, emotional beings. They are not machines, and they feel physical pain when it is inflicted on them. They are capable of experiencing a wide range of emotions, including loneliness, embarrassment, sadness, longing, depression, anxiety, panic, and fear, as well as joy, relief, surprise, happiness, contentment, and peace. At times, some may exhibit behavior that shows a highly

developed sense of morality and ethics. Animals talk to each other, and some even try to talk to us.[83] They may not speak human languages, although some primates have been taught American Sign Language; they nonetheless have highly developed communication skills and vocal languages of their own that no human being has yet mastered, except maybe Dr. Dolittle.

30. Q: I agree that factory farms are horrible, so I eat only happy meat that comes from free-range animals who have had a good life and are slaughtered humanely. Isn't that okay?

A: Let me ask you this: If you were living a happy life, would you want to die? And would you personally be okay with being murdered violently, having your throat cut, your body hung upside down by one foot until you bled to death? How do you humanely kill someone who doesn't want to die?

31. Q: I don't eat meat, but I eat fish. Isn't that all right? Isn't it true that fish are cold-blooded and don't feel pain?

A: Actually, fish are very sensitive creatures with highly developed nervous systems. They feel pain acutely. If they weren't able to feel pain, they, like us, could not have survived as a species. Their nervous systems, like ours, secrete opiate-like pain-dampening biochemicals in response to pain.[84] Here is an example that may help

83 David Shariatmadari. "These Dolphins Talk to Each Other. Why Do We Insist It Isn't Language?," *Guardian* (April 20, 2016), https://www.theguardian.com/commentisfree/2016/apr/20/dolphins-talk-language-animal-communication-cooperation

84 Pamela Rice, *10 Reasons Why I'm a Vegetarian* (New York: Lantern, 2005), 168–169.

you understand just how sensitive a fish is. If you were a fish, and you were to touch a doorknob, you would be able to *feel* the presence of every person who had touched that doorknob during the course of a day.[85] Have you seen how fish are able to swim in a school so precisely relating to their fish fellows and never clumsily bump into one another? That's because they have a highly developed sense of feeling in their bodies, which enables them to feel not only the movement of the water against their skin but also the presence of other beings who are close.

Fishing is not a benign activity; it is hunting in the water. Fish are complex beings who choose mates, use language to communicate, build nests, cooperate with one another to find food, have long-term memories, and use tools. For more information, visit www.nofishing .net or www.pisces.demon.co.uk.

32. Q: *Is it okay to drink organic milk?*
A: Cows that are fed organic food are still kept as slaves on farms, regardless of whether it is a large corporate factory farm or a small family farm. As a yoga practitioner with some understanding of how karma works, you have to ask the question "If I am seeking liberation, will it serve my purpose to rob other beings of their freedom?" We ourselves can never be free if we rob others of their freedom. Besides, every dairy cow, no matter what she has been fed, ends up in the slaughterhouse.

---

85 Peter Redgrove, *The Black Goddess and the Unseen Real* (New York: Grove, 1987), 21.

33. Q: Don't cows need to be milked? Isn't it cruel not to milk them?

A: A cow, like other female mammals (including human females), doesn't give milk unless she is pregnant or has given birth to a baby. The milk her body produces is intended to provide nourishment for her baby. In our modern dairies, calves never get to nurse from their mothers longer than a few hours. They are taken away and fed synthetic formulas laden with growth-stimulating drugs and other pharmaceuticals, while we steal the milk for ourselves. Farmers profit financially from this theft and degradation. We are the only animals who steal and drink the milk from other species.

Dr. Benjamin Spock, a leading authority on child nutrition, printed an apology in the eighth edition of his best-selling book *Baby and Child Care* for ever suggesting feeding cow's milk to babies. He also advised a vegan diet for children, writing that children can get plenty of protein and iron from vegetables, beans, and other plant foods and thus avoid the fat and cholesterol in animal products. Another leading medical authority in the field of diet, Neal Barnard, says, "To give a child animal products is a form of child abuse."[86]

---

86 Activist Facts, "Neal Barnard," Activist Facts, https://www.activistfacts.com/person/455-neal-barnard.

34. Q: Aren't cows sacred to yogis? Aren't milk and ghee considered perfect sattvic foods for a yogi?
A: The Sanskrit term *sattvic* means "good, clean, and pure" and cannot be used to describe milk products, which are not clean or pure. "Cow's milk is literally a cocktail of pus, hormones, antibiotics, pesticides, and urea," says homeopathic doctor Nandita Shah of SHARAN, the Sanctuary for Health and Reconnection to Animals and Nature in Mumbai.[87] Cow's milk may be the perfect food for calves but certainly is not good for human beings. Yoga may have originated in India, where the cow has been revered as sacred for thousands of years, but times have changed since Lord Krishna played his flute for the cows of Vrindavan. There are factory farms in India now. European cows have been inbred with the native cows of India, resulting in a short-legged breed that is no longer useful in the heavy work of pulling carts or plowing fields. This doesn't limit the ability of the cows to produce milk, but approximately half the calves born are male. What happens to all the male calves being born in dairies? Their bodies wind up in the large black market focusing on beef and the sale of other products derived from cows. India is the leading exporter of leather to America and Europe. The tanning process involved in the leather is highly toxic and maims or kills thousands of people every year. Since it is illegal in many Indian states to kill a cow, there is much denial and secrecy surrounding the exploitation of cows in India.

---

87 SHARAN, "Milk Is Not Healthy," SHARAN, https://www.sharan-india.org/milk-is-not-healthy.

— SPIRITUAL REALIZATION —

Be the change you wish to see in the world.
—MAHATMA GANDHI

*And the law says whatever you do is
going to come right back on you.*
—GEORGE HARRISON (FROM THE SONG "THE LORD
LOVES THE ONE THAT LOVES THE LORD")

**35. *Q: Human beings have always eaten meat. It's
natural; even animals eat other animals. Shouldn't
we as yogis try to live a more natural life?***
A: Some meat eaters defend meat eating by pointing out
that it is natural: In the wild, animals eat one another.
The animals that end up on our breakfast, lunch, and
dinner plates, however, aren't those who normally eat
other animals. The animals we exploit for food are not
the lions and tigers and bears of the world. We eat the
gentle vegan animals. However, on today's farms, we
actually force them to become meat eaters by making
them eat feed containing the rendered remains of other
animals, which they would never eat in the wild.

Lions and other carnivorous animals do eat meat,
but that doesn't mean we should. They would die if
they didn't eat meat. Human beings, in contrast, choose
to eat meat; it isn't a physiological necessity. In fact, we
are designed anatomically to be vegans (see question #5
under Health). Lions and other carnivorous animals do
a lot of things besides eat meat. They live outdoors, not

in houses; they don't wear clothes or drive around in cars. Why cite just one of the many things that they do and argue that we should imitate them? This doesn't make much sense.

Besides, there are many activities that human beings have been doing "forever." We might argue from that perspective that eating meat should be allowed to continue. Rape has existed for thousands of years; does that mean that it is normal and should be allowed to continue? No, human beings came to recognize rape as a crime. Yogis investigate all long-standing habits and behaviors and evaluate them by one criterion: Does this activity bring me or the world closer to enlightenment?

It is wise for the yogi to consider that when someone causes harm to another, that action perpetuates the wheel of *samsara*, the cycle of birth, life, and death. The yogi is attempting to be free of *samsara* and therefore does not eat meat, since it creates the type of karma that keeps us bound to the wheel.

36. Q: Why have human beings treated animals so poorly for so many years—enslaving, torturing, exploiting, and massacring them?
A: That is the *big* question each of us must answer for the animals and ourselves. Perhaps we have treated them so poorly because we have the means to do so and can get away with it. Perhaps in a perverted attempt to feel powerful ourselves, we exert power over others who are defenseless against our weapons of mass destruction (poisons, bombs, guns, spears, knives, forks, etc.). Perhaps, because of our unenlightenment,

we do not know that what we do to others we ultimately do to ourselves. Perhaps because of our ignorance of who we really are, we strive for a sense of identity through dominating others. Perhaps we are so unconscious about our actions that we don't even realize the immense suffering we are causing to animals, the planet, and ourselves. Perhaps we have become so addicted to our greed-driven habits that we have lost our moral compass and don't know what is right and wrong. Perhaps we have just gone along with the crowd and haven't questioned our assumptions or our behavior in regard to our fellow earthlings. Perhaps common sense is not so common.

37. *Q: Are all meat eaters bad people, all vegans good people, and all animals innocent victims?*
A: No. Everyone is caught in the web of his or her own actions and is bound by past karmas (actions). *Good* and *bad* are relative terms. Every action takes one to the next place. One's knowledge of karma should not be used to judge others. You should ask yourself, "Do I like where I am going, or do I want to change my direction?" Through yoga practice, you can change the course of your life by purifying your karma. But to do that, you must have an idea of where you've been and where you want to go. Patanjali tells us that if we practice *aparigraha*—greedlessness, the fifth yama—we will begin to understand not only where we have come from but also where we are going and how our karmas have contributed to where we are now.

38. Q: *I practice yoga and am a vegan because it makes me feel healthier. I consider myself a very physical, down-to-earth person and don't believe in karma; it sounds too New Age. Do I need to believe in karma to be a yogi?*

A: Please don't be afraid of the word *karma*. There is nothing New Age about karma. *Karma* is actually a very old Sanskrit word that simply means "action." It is not a matter of belief; action is a fact. The actions we take create reactions. Every condition can be traced back to a cause or multiple causes. The karmas, or actions, we take or have taken have made our present bodies what they are. Our bodies contain an accumulation of unresolved actions, held in our cells and tissues. All the actions we take, even subtle actions like thoughts, affect our bodies and certainly our minds and emotions. Our actions for the most part involve others. The thoughts in our minds are mainly about our relationships to others—how we think about others and how we think that others think about us. Our bodies do not lie—they portray our karmas. The practice of yoga and especially the practice of asana is the practice of resolving your karmas—in other words, improving your relationships. Certainly, the choice to eat a vegan diet improves your relationship to the animals you didn't eat as well as your relationship to the planet. The actions you are taking by practicing yoga and being vegan are allowing you to feel more comfortable and at ease in your own body, and more comfortable and at ease with the world.

39. *Q: If the law of karma is true, shouldn't we accept the fact that animals are suffering because of their karmas?*

A: It is true that every being is enjoying life or suffering as a direct result of his or her own past actions. The animals in the factory farms may have been meat-eating human beings in a previous birth; we don't know, and it is not our place to judge. Nonetheless, their suffering provides us with an opportunity to step in and alleviate suffering where we see it. By choosing to be kind instead of cruel, we can break the karmic chain of reacting to violence with more violence, contributing to a more peaceful future for everyone.

40. *Q: I want to be a regular person with a normal social life. Can I also be a yogi?*

A: Vedic wisdom states that a yogi is someone who lives his or her life according to these four beliefs: God, karma, reincarnation, and vegetarianism. The company you keep—who you associate with—will determine your ability to maintain your yogic aspirations. It is always advisable to cultivate *satsang,* association with others who remind you of your highest potential and don't keep you mired in normalcy. Yogis are not normal people, after all—they are supranormal!

41. *Q: How does mindfulness meditation help one become a better activist?*

A: Meditation brings clarity and welcomes new possibilities. It helps us let go of our obsessive thinking about what others should or should not be doing. Let others do what they feel they need to do. Stop meddling in other people's business; mind your own business. Meditation is the practice of minding your own business. I am not fond of the word *mindfulness*, because it implies being full of mind/full of thoughts. Actually, the practice of meditation is designed to free you from thoughts. It is the practice of letting go of thoughts. You watch your mind think—you sit in the place of the witness, acknowledging each thought as it comes—but you don't hold on to the thought. You let it go.

We are actors, acting out the script written by our past karmas, the actions we have done before. Most of those actions have been interactions with others, and so it is normal that our minds are filled with thoughts about others. But the practice of meditation is designed to help us transcend our personality to clear the path so as to connect to something larger, to who we really are, the indwelling eternal soul whose nature is goodness. To meditate is to participate in the phenomena of watching storm clouds of thought give way to the blue sky of the eternal soul with its infinite possibilities.

42. Q: *Veganism goes against my religion. I'm a Christian, and in the Bible, God tells us to eat animals; this is told in the story of Abraham and Isaac from Genesis. God tells Abraham to make a sacrifice of his only son, Issac. But when he is ready to kill Issac, an angel appears and stops him. Nearby is a ram caught in the bushes, so Abraham kills the ram instead.*

A: Genesis is a book found in the Old Testament part of the Bible, right? If you are a Christian, then I assume that means you follow the teachings of Jesus Christ, who came with a New Testament for us to live by, and central to those teachings are "Love thy neighbor as thyself" and "Treat others as you would want to be treated." Many references support the view that Jesus was not in favor of animal sacrifice.

It was the slaughter of animals in the name of God that led Jesus to the only aggressive confrontation reported in his ministry and ultimately gave the religious authorities reason to demand his crucifixion a few days later. That confrontation took place at the Temple of Jerusalem a few days before Passover, where Jesus took direct action and freed animals who were about to be slaughtered and offered in a sacrificial rite and in doing so attacked the economic foundation of Jerusalem, disrupting a Jewish religious procedure that had been in place for centuries.

The incident must be significant, because it is mentioned in four gospels: Matthew, Mark, Luke, and John. Matthew 21:12: "Jesus entered the temple courtyard and began to drive out all the people buying and selling animals for sacrifice. He knocked over the tables of the moneychangers and the benches of those selling doves." And in John 2.14–16: "When it was almost time for the Jewish Passover, Jesus went to Jerusalem. In the temple courtyard, he found men selling oxen, lambs, pigeons, and doves. He made a whip of cords and drove them all out of the temple, he poured out the money and overturned the tables and said, 'Do not make God's house a house of trade.'" The trade that was going on was the buying and selling of animals to be slaughtered in the temple. Most temples in the ancient world (including Vedic India) were the precursors of our modern-day slaughterhouses. At the time of this incident with Jesus, the primary activity of the Jerusalem temple during Passover and other Jewish holy days was animal sacrifice—ritualized animal slaughter. The gutters that drained from the Jerusalem temple were filled with the blood of sacrificed animals.

People would pour into Jerusalem during these holy days because the law decreed that they make their offering at the temple in the city. In the courtyard and along the streets leading up to the temple were businessmen selling animals (livestock) as well as moneychangers; if you were from an outlying province, you would first have to exchange your money for the local currency to be able to buy an animal to take it up to the temple to be killed. The fact is that the commodification of animals formed the economic foundation in the ancient world, as it still does today. What Jesus did by disrupting the trading tables was seen as radical in his time, comparable to disrupting the stock market trade on Wall Street today.

Jesus offered a new way profoundly different from the old ways of the past, which were based on fear of God and satisfying him with burnt animal offerings mediated by temple priests. Jesus offered the way of love, revealing a God of compassion who exuded concern for all creatures. I would even add that this incident shows that Jesus could be considered an animal rights activist engaging in direct action. It is ironic that with the crucifixion on Good Friday, he became the sacrificial lamb a few days after this temple incident.

43. Q: Animal sacrifice as a way to appease God is a barbaric religious practice of the ancient past. Haven't we come a long way since then?

A: It is true that many religious traditions have abandoned sacrificing animals, while others continue to do so to this day. For example, in the religion of Santeria, practiced in many Caribbean countries, the ritualized slaughter of animals continues to be a central feature.[88]

In India, mostly in places where Shaktism or goddess worship is found, animals are still killed and offered to the deity.[89] The Vedic Indians were carnivorous.[90] In ancient India, animal sacrifice was prevalent, and it is mentioned in some scriptures such as the Yajurveda. But in the fifth century BCE, primarily due to Buddhism and the resurgence of Jainism, animal sacrifice began to fade out as Hinduism adopted vegetarianism. Krishna bhakti, elucidated in scriptural texts like the Bhagavad Gita, along with important philosophical/religious texts such as Patanjali's Yoga Sutras and the Hatha Yoga Pradipika, reject animal sacrifice and promote a vegetarian diet for yogis from ethical, karmic, and spiritual points of view.

---

88 BBC, "Animal Sacrifice in Santeria," BBC, https://www.bbc.co.uk/religion/religions/santeria/ritesrituals/sacrifice.shtm.

89 Christopher John Fuller. *The Camphor Flame: Popular Hinduism and Society in India* (Princeton, NJ: Princeton University Press, 2004), 46, 83–85.

90 Alain Daniélou. *A Brief History of India* (Rochester, VT: Inner Traditions Intl. 2003), 43.

The three religions based on the tradition of God as revealed to Abraham—Judaism, Islam, and Christianity—still engage in the ritualized killing, offering, and eating of animals. Certain animals are allowed to be killed and eaten if they are slaughtered in a certain way: In Judaism, it is kosher slaughter, Islam has halal dietary laws, and many Christians sacrifice animals and eat them as part of worship on holy days like Easter and Christmas.[91]

But by far, the highest numbers of animals slaughtered (ranging in the billions every year) are sacrificed unceremoniously on the altar of trade in the global church of commerce.

44. Q: Does bhakti have a place in the life of a spiritual activist?
A: Life gives us an opportunity to remember who we really are—to reconnect to our true Self, the Divine within. This is the meaning of yoga. Yoga cannot arise if there is no love for the eternal source. To be devoted to God is to love God; this is the meaning of bhakti. What do we have in life but our actions? By offering all our actions—every thought, word, and deed—to God, we surrender those actions and thus purify those actions by relinquishing small selfish motives like fear, jealousy, and anger and in turn opening to the possibility of becoming an instrument for love and compassion. This transforms the person into someone with exalted senses able to

---

91 Rod Preece. *Animals and Nature: Cultural Myths, Cultural Realities* (Vancouver: UBC Press, 2011); Lisa Kemmerer and Anthony J. Nocella. *Call to Compassion: Religious Perspectives on Animal Advocacy* (Herndon, VA: Lantern Books, 2011).

perceive deeply into the souls of others and see God there. This type of person does not exclude anyone and is naturally gentle, kind, and a friend to all. It is said that animals seek the company of the bhakta, birds sing to them, and the trees bend low to be near as they walk through the forest.

45. Q: What does it mean to be a spiritual person?
A: All living beings are spiritual beings because all of life breathes. Breath is an indication that spirit is present. The words for *spirit* in the ancient languages of Aramaic (*ruha*) and Hebrew (*ruach*) also mean "breath." Even in English, *breath* is defined as "the vital spirit, which animates living beings." Our breath is connected to the air that *every being* breathes. By breathing consciously, we acknowledge our communion with all of life. There are atoms of air in your lungs that were once in the lungs of everyone who has ever lived. In essence, we are breathing (inspiring) one another. To be alive is to be breathing. To live and breathe with an exclusive focus on one's small self, disconnected from the whole, is the definition of egotism. The enemy of the spirit is the selfish ego, which thinks that happiness can be gained through causing unhappiness and disharmony to others. In many ancient languages, the word for *enemy* means "one who falls out of rhythm; one who is not working in harmony with the larger group."[92]

Freedom from this disharmony can begin when one lets go of the breath as "my" breath. As we let go, we

---

92 See Neil Douglas-Klotz. *The Hidden Gospel: Decoding the Spiritual Message of the Aramaic Jesus* (Wheaton, IL: Quest, 1999), 41–45.

enter into the shared life force, into a sense of harmony that connects us all: the breath, the Holy Spirit. If you want to know if someone is a "spiritual being," ask yourself, "Is he or she breathing?" If the answer is yes, you know that you are in the presence of a spiritual being.

46. Q: Can you eat meat and still be a spiritual person?
A: All breathing beings are spiritual; this includes everyone who breathes, whether they are animals or humans, carnivores or vegans.

47. Q: How can you care about animals when there is so much human suffering going on in the world?
A: For compassion to truly be compassion, it can't discriminate. Compassion has to be limitless; it has to extend to all beings. If yogis are to come to the realization of the interconnectedness of life, we must free ourselves from the conditioning that has caused us to think it is all right to exclude all the other animals from our own goals of peace, freedom, and happiness. We must stop viewing ourselves as separate and disconnected from the rest of life, as if we are a special case and the laws of nature do not apply to us. Besides, the way we treat animals is causing most of the human suffering in the world, from poverty, starvation, disease, and war to lack of clean air and water.

48. Q: Being a victim of sexual abuse myself, I am a staunch supporter of the #MeToo movement and feel

that animal rights people like you, who equate the abuse of animals to the abuse of women, are absurd and insulting and distracting us from the important issue of feminine equality.

A: I am all for feminine equality. I also feel that no one should be mistreated because of gender, race, ethnicity, religion, or species and feel that we need a wider viewpoint when it comes to respect for another's body. Our culture does not value respect for bodily sovereignty—the idea that a person's body is their body. *Respect* comes from the Latin word *respectus*, which means "look and to look again." Disrespect implies a failure to look at—to really see or to consider—the feelings and needs of another. I feel that the #MeToo movement, as well as the pro-choice movement, is forcing us all to look and to look again at how we treat women.

But I feel strongly that unless we are willing to extend our concerns to include all female beings who are victims of sexual abuse, human as well as nonhuman, we will remain a culture mired in deep-rooted prejudices that allow the right to justice, equality, and the pursuit of happiness only to a minority. If we start making exceptions and say it's not okay to rape some but it is okay to rape others, it leaves the underlying corrupt misogynistic tendencies in place. For example, in the United States, there are laws that prosecute a rapist, but those laws are lax or nonexistent if the victim is a Native American woman and the crime was committed on Native American land.

What goes on down on the farm is another example. Farms have traditionally been a place where rape and sexual abuse is commonplace. A farmer, for example, does not allow his or her cow to decide what happens to her own body. Daily, she is held in place while a farmer or a hired hand or a machine pulls at her nipples, milking her, while her own mooing objections are ignored. The bodies of animals are not respected and instead are viewed as property. Billions of animals raised for slaughter are all victims of sexual abuse, but their #MeToo voices go unheard and their suffering is mostly unseen or not acknowledged as significant. (Please see chapter 6, "Brahmacharya: Good Sex.")

These exceptions invalidate the feminist movement and keep in place the underlying misogyny existing in men as well as women. The problem with situational ethics is that they are not ethical and exceptionalism corrodes the entire argument.

49. *Q: I grew up poor and often went hungry as a kid, and for that reason, as an adult, I am thankful and eat whatever is offered to me without making a fuss like you vegan folks. Why can't you just eat what's on your plate?*
A: I grew up poor also, but I did grow up and came to understand the connection between poverty and the consumption of meat and dairy in our world.

50. *Q: Why are we violent?*
A: By definition, the ego is unable to experience compassion. Self-centered interests motivate a person whose identity is bound in the I-ness of the ego. The root cause of violence is a lack of true Self-confidence,

confidence that comes directly from God—the Supreme Self. Those who resort to violence think that by causing harm to another, they will benefit. They put their own temporary gratification above another's happiness. This is the underlying reason a person could rationalize a violent action like eating meat that involves intense violence in the enslaving, abusing, and of course the killing of the animal. But they sanction it because they think the benefit to themselves matters more than the suffering of animals or the devastation of the environment. They put their faith in the shortsighted ego, which is never satisfied and always grabbing externally. They don't look inside to the source of happiness and freedom, which is their very own soul, that which is whole and complete and needing nothing but its Self to be happy.

Spiritual activists realize that their actions matter and that how they treat others will eventually but inevitably create the future conditions for how they themselves will be treated. If happiness is your goal, do everything you can to contribute to the happiness of others. Treating others as you would want to be treated is a win/win for everyone. Let your priority shift from self-centeredness to other-centeredness. Let go of the obsession with the question "What's in it for me?" Replace it with "How can I serve others?" and "How can I enhance their lives and increase God's bliss in this world?"

51. *Q: Why do human beings aspire to be on top by controlling others?*

A: We have been conditioned to believe that the person who controls the lives of others has the most power, wealth, and influence and is thought to be successful in life. This belief rests on the assumption of the hierarchy of control and is exhibited in the bullying behavior of many, from the highest in government and corporate positions to the less influential members of our society who have only animals to kick around. This type of success does not bring happiness, as it makes for an unstable relationship with others who live in fear of you. True success can be measured by how much you are loved, not how much fear you can elicit.

52. Q. *Admittedly, exploiting animals is not a nice thing to do, but isn't it inevitable for human progress? Look at our history. Without the horse, for example, we could not have traveled or ploughed fields to plant grain. Without sheep and goats, we would not have been able to clothe ourselves when the weather got cold. And without little animals like rats, mice, rabbits, and guinea pigs, we could not have discovered medicines to cure disease.*

A: And, I might add, without human slaves, we couldn't have built the great palaces and monuments of the past or made cotton a lucrative commodity. And don't forget about the trees—without cutting down all the forests, how could we have built railroads to transport our commodities? Without commodities, we couldn't make money and perpetuate the "Might is right" idea of human supremacy and hierarchy within our societies.

What kind of progress are we talking about—the progress of greed?

When we look deeper into the causes of our present woes and miseries, we will see that the karmic retribution for our shortsighted exploitive actions toward others and the Earth is a heavy debt to pay and ultimately outweighs any temporary appearance of gain. The Yogic teachings caution about seeking prosperity and happiness by taking it from another. In the Christian tradition, we also hear the echoes of karma when Jesus says that the key to happiness is to love others as yourself and that you should treat them as you would want to be treated. In the end, profiting by hurting others never yields a truly satisfying profit.

53. *Q: Based on the current situation in the world, why should we want to become vegans and spiritual activists? It seems like the passive approach. Isn't more direct action needed? Shouldn't we get rid of the corrupt politicians and greedy corporate leaders?*
A: The world is a reflection of us—our own minds turned inside out and providing a mirror image back to us. We cannot change the world externally by blaming, complaining, and pointing fingers and insisting that other people should do this or that. Finding fault with others and seeking ways to rid them from our world will result in disappointment, frustration, and anger. Change must come from within. We can work on changing ourselves internally by rooting out the negative traits within ourselves we see others exhibiting. If we see suffering, evil, cruelty, injustice, etc., in the world and we want it

to change, the most direct means is to change ourselves and not insist that the world, or other people, change. Can we root out the evil, the cruelty, the injustice in ourselves? It is up to us to change; the world will follow.

54. Q: How do you feel about the exploitation of yoga as a vehicle for profit, especially when the principle of ahimsa is usually completely disregarded?
A: Like everything in life, yoga appears according to how you see it. Yoga is immense and not easily comprehended in its totality, like the elephant in the ancient story of the blind men who were asked what an elephant is. The one who was holding the tail said, "An elephant is long and stiff like a rope." The man who was holding a leg said, "An elephant is solid and heavy like an old tree." The one who was touching the ear said, "An elephant is delicate and thin like a leaf." And on it goes. Patanjali describes this phenomena in the following yoga sutra:

---

vastu-sāmye citta-bhedāt tayor vibhaktaḥ panthāḥ
PYS IV.15

*Each individual person perceives the same object in
a different way, according to their own state of mind
and projections. Everything is empty from its own
side and appears according to how you see it.*

The yoga that you practice might not be the yoga that I practice. The yoga of 2,000 years ago is not the same as the yoga of today, and the yoga 2,000 years from now will not be the same as today or yesterday.

So, the point is that yoga is adaptable to each person and to each age. It yields its teachings in a way that the mind can grasp it. Yoga's mercurial nature allows it to move according to what's needed or what's asked for. Nonetheless, the universal essential nature of Yoga as enlightenment is always available to those who wish to embrace the practices of yoga as transformational, magical, and alchemical.

Our present culture is predominantly a materialistic one. Money, and the material things it can buy, is held in the highest esteem. The actions of most human beings are motivated by money. A person will contemplate whether to do something according to how much money it costs or how much he or she might get from the venture. Freedom is equated with the ability to buy; shopping is valued highly and given the status of a human right. I think that one of the reasons we treat animals so badly is because they have no money; we treat children badly for the same reason, but we don't eat them. Why? Perhaps because our children will grow up to be shoppers and animals won't.

55. Q: How do I become a vegan?

A: You could begin gradually by, for example, being vegan one day a week. Choose a day, and on that day, don't eat any meat, milk, eggs, or fish. This would make a big difference to your health, to the environment, and to the animals spared. Alternatively, you can try giving up meat and dairy foods one at a time, quitting milk, fish, eggs, or meat, etc. Remember that you are not inflicting punishment on or depriving yourself, but rather fostering a longer, happier, healthier life for you and the planet. Or just immediately stop participating in the cruelty; just stop, period. Why, if you know the truth about how animals are treated, would you want to eat them ever again? The truth shall set you free. The door of your cage is open; just walk out. Why not go for it? Be totally free. Leave the cage forever and never go back.

56. *Q: How can I be an effective speaker and use my words to move people to be more compassionate toward animals and stop eating them?*

A: Be a joyful vegan yourself. View everyone as providing you with opportunities to be kind and to articulate empathy and compassion for another being. See whomever you speak to as a holy being. Do not see anyone as mean, stupid, or compassionless or as a person who needs you to enlighten him or her. If you can't see people you speak to as compassionate, how can you ever expect them to see themselves that way?

Before you speak to someone, ask yourself, *How do I want this person to feel about himself or herself?* Do you have the largeness of heart to see that person's highest potential? For that to occur, you must be willing to give up any negative thoughts about him or her in order to provide a space for the person to turn around in. Keep in mind that when you are speaking to others, they can always *feel* your underlying contempt or respect for them, and that will determine whether they are able to hear your message. What is your goal in speaking to them? Is it to vent your anger, to assert your superiority, to berate them, or to make them feel guilty? Or do you really want to empower them to change for the better and to become the kind of people who don't cause animals to suffer? If you really want them to stop eating meat, you must see in them the potential to do that, and you must speak to that potential.

57. Q: What is the biggest misconception about spiritual activism you have experienced so far?
A: When it is thought that hate and anger are more powerful motivators than love and acceptance. When you think the world is out there coming at you and you have to fight back, you are engaged in war, and war never brings peace and cannot activate the inner force of love within you. To separate the world into vegans and meat eaters, good guys and bad guys, or victims and perpetrators will result only in more division, not the peaceful unification we seek as spiritual activists.

The misconception about activism in general starts with a confusion about the effectiveness of advocacy without aggression. Aggression is confrontational and *against*, whereas advocacy is *for*. There is a misconception that advocacy expressed without aggression will be perceived as too touchy-feely and ineffective, whereas advocacy linked with aggression is commonly regarded as more effective. This idea that you need to be aggressive to effectively get your point across and thus elicit change undermines any chance for communication, and without communication, intelligent solutions to problems become impossible. You can't make lasting effective change through merely expressing your anger. Advocacy with a long-term aim forces you to look deeper into the issue and come up with solutions for all involved. It takes two people to make a fight; it takes one to make a difference.

The ability to find common ground to begin a conversation is essential. For that to happen, you have to let go of any animosity or contempt you may feel toward the other person. Aggression, as well as advocacy, can come in the form of actions, words, and thoughts. Thoughts are the precursor to words and actions. A person can always feel how you feel about them, and this will determine the outcome of any interaction. Again, if you can't see others as potentially kind and compassionate beings, how can you ever expect them to see themselves that way?

To think well of another and to want that person's happiness, even though you do not agree with the person's current thoughts and actions, is the key to spiritual activism.

When you engage in conversation with others who may not agree with your point of view, be sure that you are coming from a place of tolerance yourself. "I try to treat whomever I meet as an old friend," says the Dalai Lama. "This gives me a genuine feeling of happiness— this is the practice of compassion. A truly compassionate attitude towards others does not change even if they are behaving negatively." And from Harvard professor Arthur C. Brooks, "When you feel contempt for another person, practice warmheartedness towards them."[93] Dr. Martin Luther King Jr. put it this way: "You have no moral grounding with someone who can feel your underlying contempt for them."

58. *Q: Do you think everyone should be vegan?*
A: No, because everyone is not, although if human beings were to become vegan, we would all benefit. Even though I have been a vegan and a yogi for most of my life, I don't feel it is up to me to tell others what they should or should not do. It is up to each person to make his or her own choices. It seems that most of us make better choices when we are well informed, so if someone is interested and asks me a question about veganism or yoga, I welcome the opportunity to engage in conversation and will gladly do my best to share what I have discovered.

---

93 Arthur C. Brooks, https://arthurbrooks.com.

CHAPTER 13

YOGA
ON THE MAT

YOGA ASANA IS A CONSCIOUS SPIRITUAL PRACTICE—A sadhana that can purify and resolve our relationships with others as we take the practice of the yamas into our experience on the mat. The practice of asana can purify one's perception of oneself and others and lead to enlightenment, which is the realization of the oneness of being.

Enlightened yogis know that they are not the body nor the mind; rather, they "have" bodies and minds. The true Self is eternal. It can be challenging to realize that, however. Our bodies are made of our past karmas, which propel us into the experience of birth, which, in turn, is our opportunity to live and to realize who we really are beyond the vehicle that is the body/mind container.

Asana means "seat," and *seat* means "connection to the Earth." Earth implies all beings and things. *Chakra* means "wheel." A chakra is a doorway through which we perceive reality. Our ability to see into the various dimensions of reality is reflected in the energetic ease or "dis-ease" found in our relationships. The disease of feeling disconnected from oneself and others is pervasive in our time. This disconnection causes us to hurt and exploit others, which results only in unhappiness and disease for others as well as ourselves.

Each asana corresponds to a specific chakra, as well as to a specific relationship. The practice of asana is a practical method for purifying our relationships, ultimately revealing to us our true nature as not separate, but as interconnected with all beings.

Karma means "action" and includes every thought, word, and deed we have done. The fact is, we do not act alone—our thoughts, words, and deeds are done in relation to others. Our karmas bind us to our relationships with others. Because our bodies are made of our past karmas, every asana provides an opportunity to access and heal these relationships. The purification of our relationships brings about a healing of the disease of disconnection and the reestablishment of a sound body and sound mind, able to embody, radiate, and communicate peace and joy to all.

If you preface your asana practice with the intention to resolve past relationships, then, while you are in each asana, allow the experience to help you remember those past relationships. If pain, doubt, or tightness arise, give silent blessings to the others in your life. The following descriptions might help you reflect on the power of asana practice to heal relationships by resolving them into love, forgiveness, and blessing while on the mat.

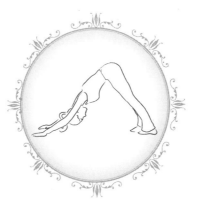

1st Chakra: MULADHARA

(Root Place)
Standing Asanas

Karmic relationships:
Mother Earth, nature, parents, home,
job, money, boss, workplace

Your spiritual journey begins with acknowledging your physicality through devotion to the Great Goddess, Mother Nature. If you cannot be at peace with your parents and feel contentment with your body, home, and job, you won't be able to evolve. You purify the foundation by seeing all of life as sacred. Your connection to the Earth must be based in steadiness and joy not only for yourself but also for the whole world and all beings.

The practice of standing asanas develops stability and removes fear.

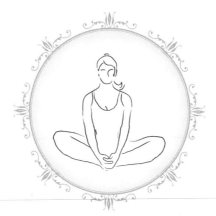

2nd Chakra: SWADHISHTHANA

(Her Favorite Standing Place)
Forward Bends

Karmic relationships:
Creative, artistic, romantic, and sexual partners

You can purify your creative/sexual relationships by letting go of anger, blame, and resentment. Through practice, you will come to realize that the way others treat you is coming from how you have treated others in your past. Forward bending takes you into your past with an opportunity to reflect and heal through letting go of resentful feelings you may be holding against past partners.

 The practice of forward bending develops creativity and removes sorrow and envy.

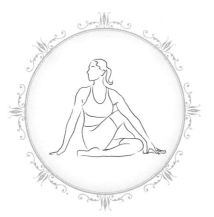

3rd Chakra: MANIPURA

(Jewel in the City)
Twists

Karmic relationships:
Others you have hurt (especially focus on animals
you may have eaten or caused to be harmed)

Twisting asanas provide a great opportunity to reflect on the food you have eaten and the other animal beings you may have harmed in the process. Acknowledge your unwitting selfishness and ask for forgiveness. Don't feel guilty. What you have already done in your past is done; you cannot change that, but you can move forward in a new and more compassionate way, starting now. Realize that when you hurt others, it is coming from a lack of self-confidence. This practice provides the means to remedy that.

The practice of twists develops confidence and
removes anger.

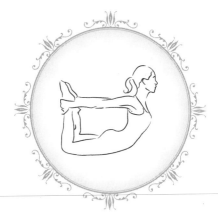

4th Chakra: ANAHATA

(Unstruck)
Backbends

Karmic relationships:
Others who have hurt you

Have the largeness of heart to let go, forgive others, and move on. Know that others, just like you, are only doing the best they can in any given situation. Backbends allow you to move into the future. The ease that you have in moving into your future will be reflected in the ease you have with forgiving others.

The practice of backbending develops compassion and forgiveness and removes hate and hostility.

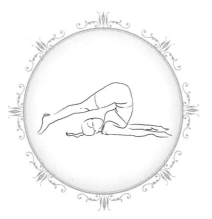

5th Chakra: VISHUDDHA

(Poison Removing)
Shoulderstand, Plough, Fish

Karmic relationship:
Yourself

Purification of this chakra helps you develop satya, purity of speech, allowing you to say what you mean and mean what you say. It enables you to see yourself as a holy being able to uplift the lives of others. If you are to attain enlightenment, you must begin to see yourself as deserving. When you vow to attain enlightenment so that you may contribute to the happiness and liberation of others, you will be freed of arrogance and cynicism in connection to your own self-image.

The practice of shoulderstand develops the ability to communicate and removes cynicism.

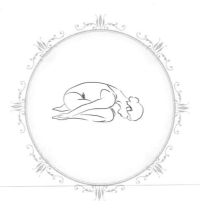

6th Chakra: AJNA

(Command Center)
Child's Seat

Karmic relationship:
Teachers

When you bow to another as your teacher, the potent elixir of humility purifies you, releasing you from selfishness, jealousy, and pride. You are then no longer attached to ego. A truly holy being is a humble being. Guru means "the enlightenment principle," and it operates through your teachers. When you see your teachers as holy, you tap into the power that can uplift the world!

The practice of child's seat develops humility and removes doubt.

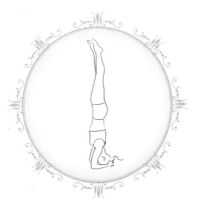

7th Chakra: SAHASRARA

(Thousand-Petaled Lotus)
Headstand

Karmic relationship:
God, the Divine or Higher Self

What is realized in the yogic state of samadhi is the oneness of being, the sacred unity of all. Separateness is transcended as the light of Divine Love reveals the cosmic unity between the individual, nature, and God.

The practice of headstand can lead to the development of enlightenment and remove disconnection.

EPILOGUE

*Blame keeps the sad game going. It keeps stealing
all your wealth—giving it to an imbecile with
no financial skills. Dear one, wise up.*

—Hafiz

YOGA IS NOT FOR EVERYONE. YOGA IS FOR THOSE WHO want to be free and believe that *moksha* is possible. Not everyone wants to be free or even recognizes that they are in bondage. Not everyone realizes that through their own actions, they could have an influence on their own freedom and on the freedom of others. What others do is not ours to judge. Remember that they, like you, are only doing the best they can. When you point a blaming finger at someone else, keep in mind that there are three other fingers pointing back at you. Our work is the work on ourselves. We must embody what we feel is good and beautiful and not wait for others to lead us.

Anyone who comes to the practice of yoga at this time in the history of the world is not a beginner. To even have an interest in these ancient liberation and devotional practices is evidence of many lifetimes of previous practice. To be able to begin to comprehend the immensity yoga offers, a person must already have some eligibility arising from past life experiences. A yogi is born with the desire to be free. Therefore, yoga

should not be proselytized. The missionary approach of converting the "ignorant savages" will not work when it comes to yoga. Trying to force people to "do" yoga because it is good for them or good for the planet is a ludicrous idea.

There is a growing number of yoga practitioners in the world today. We are incredibly privileged to be exposed to these ancient wisdom teachings and methods, which offer techniques for using compassion and kindness to bring about happiness and liberation. Human beings may have caused the present global crisis, but its disastrous consequences need not become a reality. Our actions now will greatly impact the future of our planet.

Liberation is not for everyone, but it may be for you. Yoga teaches the truth through direct experience, and the truth will set you free. Now the cage door is open, but no one will force us to walk out and leave our prison. The choice is ours alone. It is up to us and always has been. It is indeed possible for us to break the chains that bind us to the wheel of *samsara*. Whatever we want in life, we should first provide it for others. Through an understanding of how karma works, we come to realize the great impact of our own actions on the world. We realize that the bondage and suffering we experience in the world is caused by the bondage and suffering we inflict upon others. To liberate others is to liberate oneself.

Our relationship to animals is our relationship to nature. When we cease to enslave animals and cease to view them as exploitable, we break the chains of conditioning that have held us for thousands of years. As we become kinder, the world will become a kinder place. When we say no to feeding on the meat, milk, and blood of others, we say yes to liberation. We become liberated as spiritual beings, feeling a connection and sense of belonging to the living scheme of things. We experience the all-pervading divine creative presence underlying the force of nature. This allows us to let divine wisdom guide our participation in the greater unfolding of grace.

Through the awakening of humility, compassion will arise and love will be felt within our hearts. Not a mundane love, but a love supreme—God's great love. With that great love all is possible.

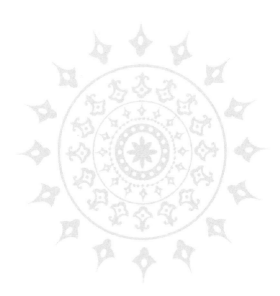

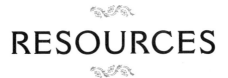

RESOURCES

Books

- *101 Reasons Why I'm a Vegetarian*, by Pamela Rice
- *Animal Liberation: A New Ethics for Our Treatment of Animals*, by Peter Singer
- *Animals as Persons: Essays on the Abolition of Animal Exploitation*, by Gary Francione
- *An Unnatural Order: Why We Are Destroying the Planet and Each Other*, by Jim Mason
- *Battered Birds, Crated Herds; How We Treat the Animals We Eat*, by Gene Bauston
- *Becoming Vegan: The Complete Reference to Plant-Based Nutrition*, by Brenda Davis, RD, and Vesanto Melina, MS, RD
- *Breaking the Food Seduction: The Hidden Reasons Behind Food Cravings—and 7 Steps to End Them Naturally*, by Neal Barnard, MD
- *Crazy Sexy Cancer*, by Kris Carr
- *Crazy Sexy Kitchen*, by Kris Carr
- *Diet for a New America: How Your Food Choices Affect Your Health, Happiness, and the Future of Life on Earth*, by John Robbins
- *Dominion: The Power of Man, the Suffering of Animals, and the Call to Mercy*, by Matthew Scully
- *Empty Cages: Facing the Challenge of Animal Rights*, by Tom Regan
- *Eternal Treblinka: Our Treatment of Animals and the Holocaust*, by Charles Patterson
- *Farm Sanctuary: Changing Hearts and Minds About Animals and Food*, by Gene Baur
- *Green Yoga*, by Georg and Brenda Feuerstein
- *Gods of Love and Ecstasy: The Traditions of Shiva and Dionysus*, by Alain Daniélou

RESOURCES

- *Hope's Edge: The Next Diet for a Small Planet*, by Frances Moore Lappé and Anna Lappé

- *Living Among Meat Eaters: The Vegetarian's Survival Handbook*, by Carol J. Adams

- *Living the Farm Sanctuary Life: The Ultimate Guide to Eating Mindfully, Living Longer, and Feeling Better Every Day*, by Gene Baur and Gene Stone

- *Mad Cowboy: Plain Truth from the Cattle Rancher Who Won't Eat Meat*, by Howard F. Lyman and Glen Merzer

- *Main Street Vegan: Everything You Need to Know to Eat Healthfully and Compassionately in the Real World*, by Victoria Moran

- *Making Kind Choices: Everyday Ways to Enhance Your Life Through Earth- and Animal-Friendly Living*, by Ingrid Newkirk

- *Meatonomics: How the Rigged Economics of Meat and Dairy Make You Consume Too Much—and How to Eat Better, Live Longer, and Spend Smarter*, by David Robinson Simon

- *One Can Make a Difference*, by Ingrid Newkirk and Jane Ratcliffe

- *Peace to All Beings: Veggie Soup for the Chicken's Soul*, by Judy Carman

- *Protest Kitchen: Fight Injustice, Save the Planet, and Fuel Your Resistance One Meal at a Time*, by Carol J. Adams and Virginia Messina

- *Seeds of Deception: Exposing Industry and Government Lies About the Safety of the Genetically Engineered Food You're Eating*, by Jeffrey M. Smith

- *Skinny Bitch: A No-Nonsense, Tough-Love Guide for Savvy Girls Who Want to Stop Eating Crap and Look Fabulous*, by Rory Freedman and Kim Barnouin

- *Slaughterhouse: The Shocking Story of Greed, Neglect, and Inhuman Treatment Inside the U.S. Meat Industry*, by Gail A. Eisnitz

- *Strolling with Our Kin: Speaking for and Respecting Voiceless Animals*, by Marc Bekoff

- *Thanking the Monkey: Rethinking the Way We Treat Animals*, by Karen Dawn

❦ *The China Study: The Most Comprehensive Study of Nutrition and the Startling Implications for Diet, Weight Loss, and Long-Term Health,* by T. Colin Campbell, PhD, and Thomas M. Campbell II, MD

❦ *The Food Revolution: How Your Diet Can Help Save Your Life and Our World,* by John Robbins

❦ *The Good Karma Diet: Eat Gently, Feel Amazing, Age in Slow Motion,* by Victoria Moran

❦ *The Inner Art of Vegetarianism: Spiritual Practices for Body and Soul,* by Carol J. Adams

❦ *The Sexual Politics of Meat: A Feminist-Vegetarian Critical Theory,* by Carol J. Adams

❦ *The Textbook of Yoga Psychology: The Definitive Translation and Interpretation of Patanjali's Yoga Sutras for Meaningful Application in All Modern Psychologic Disciplines,* by Shri Brahmananda Sarasvati

❦ *The World Peace Diet: Eating for Spiritual Health and Social Harmony,* by Will Tuttle, PhD

❦ *World Peace Yoga: Yoga for People Who Breathe,* by Anna Ferguson

❦ *Your Right to Know: Genetic Engineering and the Secret Changes in Your Food,* by Andrew Kimbrell

Films

❦ *A Prayer for Compassion*

❦ *Chew on This*

❦ *Cow*

❦ *Cowspiracy: The Sustainability Secret*

❦ *Cowspiritual*

❦ *Dominion*

❦ *Earthlings*

❦ *Forks Over Knives*

❦ *I Am an Animal*

❦ *Meet Your Meat*

❦ *Okja*

❦ *Peaceable Kingdom*

❦ *The Animals Film*

❦ *The Game Changers*

❦ *The Witness*

❦ *What Is Real? The Story of Jivamukti Yoga*

❦ *What the Health*

Organizations

❦ Animal Equality: www.animalequality.org

❦ Animal Rahat: www.animalrahat.com

❦ Animal Rights: The Abolitionist Approach:
www.abolitionistapproach.com

❦ Anonymous for the Voiceless: www.anonymousforthevoiceless.org

❦ DawnWatch media reports: www.dawnwatch.com

❦ Farm Sanctuary: www.farmsanctuary.org

❦ HappyCow: www.happycow.net

❦ Humane Society of the United States: www.hsus.org

❦ Jivamukti Yoga: www.jivamuktiyoga.com

❦ LiveKindly: www.livekindly.co

❦ Mercy for Animals: www.mercyforanimals.org

❦ PETA: www.peta.org

❦ Physicians Committee for Responsible Medicine: www.pcrm.org

❦ The Vegan Society: www.vegansociety.com

❦ Your Daily Vegan: www.yourdailyvegan.com

❦ Vegan.com: www.vegan.com

❦ Vegan Outreach: www.veganoutreach.org

❦ VegNews: www.vegnews.com

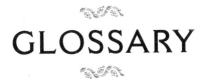

GLOSSARY

abhinivesha: excessive fear of death, one of the five *kleshas*, or obstacles to Self-realization

abhyasa: *as* (to throw) + *abhi* (toward): to throw oneself into something; steady continuous practice; repeated endeavor. Abhyasa leads to spiritual development and wisdom.

abolitionist: someone who wants to abolish, or do away with, slavery

ahimsa: *a* (not) + *himsa* (harming): the practice of nonharming or nonviolence

animal: from the Latin *animalis*, meaning having a soul, one who breathes, or a living being. Humans are one animal species among many.

antu: may it be so

aparigraha: greedlessness

asana: seat; the practice of connecting well to the Earth and all beings

asmita: identification with ego or personality self; one of the five kleshas, or obstacles to Self-realization

asteya: nonstealing

avidya: ignorance; mistaking oneself, others, or reality for what it is not; perceiving reality as existing as other or separate from oneself; unenlightened thinking that you are an individual who exists disconnected from the whole—not holy; one of the five kleshas, or obstacles to Self-realization

Bhagavad Gita: The Song of the Lord. It is part of a larger work, the Mahabharata, composed by the sage Vyasa, in which Krishna explains to the warrior Arjuna the methods for attaining Yoga. Alongside Patanjali's Yoga Sutras and the Hatha Yoga Pradipika, the Gita is the essential reference book for the practices of yoga. Although scholars debate when it was written, most agree that it dates to about 200 BCE.

bhakti: loving devotion to God

bhav: the Divine mood of unity; feeling holy—connected to the whole

brahmacharya: *brahma* (Hindu god of creativity, or the creative power of becoming) + *charya* (vehicle, or a means to move or reach toward): continence, or the ability to specifically direct sexual energy toward spiritual awakening; not using sex selfishly to manipulate others

dharana: concentration; the practice of taking the mind from a fragmented disconnected state to a place of focus and wholeness; the necessary prerequisite to meditation

dharma: support; fix in place; that which holds together

genetically modified organisms (GMOs): organisms with genes that have been manipulated and altered. Human beings are genetically modifying both plants and animals, causing mutations to occur in the name of profit. No real benefit to human health or to animals, plants, or the ecosystem has resulted from this practice.

hatha yoga: uniting or joining the sun and the moon, which represent self and other

himsic: harmful

Holy Scriptures: channeled words of wisdom intended to provide inspiration and guidance to spiritual aspirants, written by rishis and sages; some examples are the Bible, the Koran, the Vedas, the Upanishads, the Yoga Sutras, the Hatha Yoga Pradipika, and the Bhagavad Gita

kirtan: praise; singing the names of God in a call-and-response manner. Kirtan as a practice "cuts" through the thinking mind.

klesha: hindrance; obstacle. Patanjali lists five kleshas to the attainment of Yoga: *avidya* (ignorance), *asmita* (egoism), *raga* (attachment to what you like), *dvesha* (aversion to what you don't like), and *abhinivesha* (fear of death).

lokah: location

jiva: individual soul

jivanmukta: a liberated soul

jivanmukti: the state of liberation

memes (pronounced "meems"): the blueprints of a civilization, culture, or way of living that become implanted in the minds of each member of that culture and remain there unquestioned, becoming "mainstream" ideology

moksha: liberation

mukti: liberation; freedom from avidya

Patanjali: a philosopher sage, considered an incarnation of the divine serpent, Sesha, who fell (pat) from heaven into the palm (anjali) of a saintly woman named Gonika. He compiled the philosophy of Yoga into terse statements (sutras), organizing them into four chapters (padas), known as the Yoga Sutras of Patanjali. There are speculations as to when he lived ranging from 5,000 BC to 300 BC.

pranayama: to control the life force in order to expand or set it free; the fourth of the eight-limbed Ashtanga method of Yoga as outlined by Patanjali

pratishthayam: to be well established or grounded in a certain practice; the result of abhyasa

Raja yoga: yoga for the king; the yoga system outlined by the eight limbs of Ashtanga yoga [*ashta* (eight) + *anga* (limb or attachment)]

satsang: *sat* (truth) + *anga* (limb or attachment): association with and attachment to the truth

tantra: *tan* (to stretch) + *tra* (to cross over): various techniques or methods used to stretch or expand consciousness, enabling one to cross over avidya

sadhana: conscious spiritual practice

samadhi: *sam* (same) + *adhi* (highest): enlightenment; ecstasy; perfect absorption; Yoga

samsara: *sam* (same) + *sara* (agitation): to be repeatedly agitated; the cycle of rebirth

satya: truthfulness

sattvic: pure; balanced; clear

shunyata: emptiness; void; lacking qualities of its own. It is equated with the feminine principle, referring to that which is vast and boundless in its potential. Reality is empty and appears according to how the seer sees it. How the seer sees it is dependent on his or her own karmas.

siddhi: power or extraordinary skill that arises through the practice of yoga

speciesism: the prejudice against nonhuman animals. The human-held belief that all other animal species are inferior. Speciesist thinking involves considering nonhuman animals—who have their own desires, needs, and complex lives—as a means to human ends. This supremacist line of "reasoning" is used to defend treating other living, feeling beings as property, objects, or even ingredients. It's a bias rooted in denying others their own agency, interests, and self-worth, often for personal materialist gain.

sukha: good space; centered in happiness; joy; freedom from suffering

sutra: thread; a succinct, terse statement

vinyasa: *vi* (ordered placement) + *nyasa* (to place on purpose in a special way in a sequence): acting consciously or mindfully in each moment of time so that the sequence of actions leads to the desired outcome; a way of practicing yoga asanas in which a sequential, ordered placement is linked with conscious breath and intention designed to bring about *nirodha*, the cessation of the fluctuations of the mind

viveka: discriminating wisdom; the ability to know what is real, true, or eternal and what is unreal, false, or impermanent

yama: restriction

Yoga: the state of enlightenment; samadhi; ecstasy; the realization of the oneness of being and the dissolving of separateness

yoga: the practices done in order to attain enlightenment or to realize the oneness of being

ACKNOWLEDGMENTS

To Victor Schonfeld and Myriam Alaux, the makers of the documentary that changed my life and put me on the path of animal activism and veganism, *The Animals Film*, and to Robert Wyatt, who composed the film's soundtrack. To Raoul Goff, Phillip Jones, Vanessa Lopez, Rachel Anderson, Lisa Fitzpatrick, Arjuna van der Kooij, Brenda Knight, Mary Teruel, and Lucy Kee of Mandala Publishing for the courage to continuously strive to provide us with books that truly enrich our lives, and for giving me the opportunity to write this one. My appreciation goes to Paul Gopal Steinberg, Lois Laxmi Hill, Jaimie Epstein, Vallabhdas, and Banka for stepping in at the last minute not only to help me straighten out my footnote issues but also to proof the text and provide meticulous copy edits to the first edition. A million thanks to the following special people for orchestrating the foreign language translations of *Yoga and Vegetarianism*: Paloma Baker: Spanish; Elena Benvenuti: Italian; Michi Kern: German; Andy C. Lin: Chinese; Heeki Park: Japanese; Yeliz Utku Konca: Turkish; and Ellen Verbeek: Russian.

Immense gratitude to Karoline Straubinger for helping on many levels to bring the 2020 revised edition to completion. Appreciation to Hari Mulukutla for his assistance in proofreading the Sanskrit sutras and in facilitating the audio recording of this book. Many thanks to my literary agent, Joel Gotler, and the many ways that he comes to my aid. To David Life for listening to me read out loud the manuscript during its many stages and providing valuable insights, as well as continuous emotional and technical support. To my holy teachers, Shri Brahmananda Sarasvati, Swami Nirmalananda, Sri K. Pattabhi Jois, Shyamdas, and Shri Milanbaba Goswami, who have taught me the value of Sanskrit and continue to teach me the meaning and value of compassion and, most importantly, bhakti.

I am in awe of and am continuously grateful to the growing number of Jivamukti Yoga teachers who have embraced animal rights and find clever as well as courageous ways to bring the message of veganism into the classes they teach all over the world. Special kudos to Jivamukti Yoga teachers Kip Andersen, Michi Kern, Rima Rabbath, Manizeh Rimer, Yeliz Utku Konca, and Beth Watson for sharing their transformational vegan stories in this book. My sincere appreciation to our fearless Jivamukti Yoga global leaders, Camilla Veen and Hari Mulukutla, for both holding our community together and radiating the authentic teachings of yoga into the world.

A very special acknowledgment to Ingrid Newkirk, my dear friend, inspiration, and co-conspirator, who in a relatively short time has managed, against all odds, to make this world a kinder place for all inhabitants. To my friends and fellow activists who inspire me to continue to be radical and speak up for the animals, even when faced with ridicule, attack, and violent opposition: Carol J. Adams, Dr. Neal Barnard, Gene Baur, Jenny Brown,

Kris Carr, Seane Corn, Chloe Jo Davis, Michael Franti, Anna Ferguson, Rory Freedman, Kathy Freston, Julia Butterfly Hill, Howard F. Lyman, Jim Mason, Victoria Moran, Jannette Patterson, Janet Rienstra-Peak, Gretchen Primack, John Robbins, Martin Rowe, Matthew Scully, Russell Simmons, Kathy Stevens, H. H. Shri Radhanath Swami, Doug Swenson, Karo Tak, Will Tuttle, and Paul Watson.

I want to acknowledge the work of Jim Mason, who wrote *An Unnatural Order: Why We Are Destroying the Planet and Each Other*, and Will Tuttle, author of *The World Peace Diet: Eating for Spiritual Health and Social Harmony*. If you found my book to be helpful, I encourage you to read their books, as they go deeper into the historical aspects of our culture's attitude toward animals and nature.

Thank you, Karen Dawn; if it wasn't for you sending me good news stories through your organization, DawnWatch.com, I would go uninformed and uninspired. I highly recommend signing up for DawnWatch Media Alerts, as they will keep you motivated and optimistic.

I want to acknowledge two great contemporary spiritual leaders of the Krishna bhakti yoga tradition: H. H. Radhanath Swami, representing the lineage of Shri Chaitanya through ISKCON, and H. H. Shri Milan Goswami, representing the Pushti Marg lineage of Shri Vallabhacharya, for their endorsements of the radical vegan message of this book.

Most important, I wish to acknowledge all the animals I have hurt in my past. I apologize for my ignorance and the ignorance of my species and hope that with this book, we can begin to heal the many wounds we have inflicted on all of you: members of the animal nations, our fellow Earthlings with whom we share life on this planet.

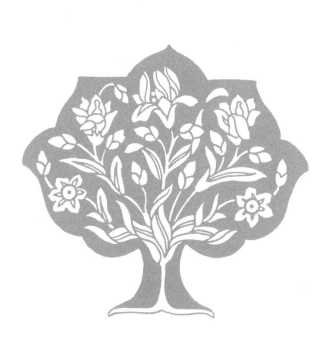

ABOUT THE AUTHOR

Sharon Gannon is changing the way people view spirituality, life, themselves, one another, animals, and the environment. Along with David Life, she is the creator of the Jivamukti Yoga method, a path to enlightenment through compassion for all beings. Blessed by her teachers, Shri Brahmananda Sarasvati, Swami Nirmalananda, Sri K. Pattabhi Jois, Shyamdas, and Shri Milan Goswami, she is a pioneer in teaching yoga as spiritual activism. Veganism is a core principle of the Jivamukti Yoga method.

The Jivamukti method has been recognized as one of the nine forms of hatha yoga practiced in the world today. *Yoga Journal* magazine has called her an innovator, and *Vanity Fair* gives her credit for making yoga cool and hip.

Gannon has authored many books and produced numerous yoga-related DVDs and music CDs. She is the recipient of the 2008 Compassionate Living Award and the 2013 PETA Compassionate Action Award. She resides in a wild forest sanctuary in upstate New York.

For more information about the author, visit jivamuktiyoga.com and simplerecipesforjoy.com.

INDEX